DATE DUE

FE 19 '97			
MR 07 '97			
MR 27 '97			
7-6-98			
JE 22 '98			
4-19-99			
5-11-99			
MY 03 '99			
SE 26 '01			
OC 09 '01			
SE 27 '01			

Demco, Inc. 38-293

A
DOSE
OF
SANITY

Also by the Author

Help for the Hyperactive Child
Psychiatric Signs and Symptoms Due to Medical Problems

A DOSE OF SANITY

MIND, MEDICINE, AND MISDIAGNOSIS

Sydney Walker III, M.D.

John Wiley & Sons, Inc.
New York • Chichester • Brisbane • Toronto • Singapore

Library of Congress Cataloging-in-Publication Data

Walker, Sydney.
    A dose of sanity : mind, medicine, and misdiagnosis / by Sydney
Walker III.
        p.   cm.
    Includes bibliographical references and index.
    ISBN 0-471-14136-4 (cloth : alk. paper)
    1. Psychological manifestations of general diseases. 2. Mental
illness—Physiological aspects. 3. Diagnostic errors.
4. Psychiatric errors. 5. Consumer education. I. Title.
    [DNLM: 1. Mental Disorders—diagnosis. 2. Diagnostic
Errors.   WM 141 W184d 1996]
RC455.4.B5W35 1996
616.89'075—dc20
DNLM/DLC
for Library of Congress   95-46671

Printed in the United States of America
10 9 8 7 6 5 4 3 2 1

To Songmin, my gracious wife,
whose support and encouragement,
through thick and thin, have made me
singularly fortunate.

Preface

I've spent over thirty years in medical practice, as both a neurologist and a psychiatrist. I've also trained in neurosurgery, and have received advanced degrees in physiology and pharmacology (the study of drugs and their effects on the body). In addition, in my formative years, I had the good fortune to be influenced by two giants: the great Derek Denny-Brown, at Harvard Medical School, and the equally renowned Sir Francis Walshe at National Hospital in Queen's Square, London.

But my best teachers have been my patients, who brought my textbook learning to life. In the course of my career, I've experienced the pleasure of seeing suicidal patients restored to happiness, hyperactive children transformed into honor-roll students, and angry or frightened or psychotic patients returned to health and independence. I've learned firsthand that a correct diagnosis, and proper treatment, can change lives—and often save them.

Unfortunately, correct diagnosis and treatment have become all too rare in psychiatry today. Far too many patients—perhaps the majority—are simply being labeled as "hyperactive," or "depressed," or "anxious," and then handed prescriptions for drugs that mask symptoms rather than treat disease. Others are being referred to psychotherapists, whose therapies, while helpful in limited ways, cannot cure brain dysfunction.

Why has this happened? Because psychiatry has become almost completely dependent on one manual, the *Diagnostic and Statistical Manual* (DSM), a "cookbook" listing of symptoms that has replaced the science of deductive differential diagnosis. Many psychiatrists use DSM to "diagnose" patients after only a cursory examination (or even no examination at all) and a handful of lab tests. But *a DSM label is not a diagnosis*—and psychiatric patients whose disorders are caused by tumors, infections, toxic exposure, hormonal imbalances, or other physical ailments will suffer needlessly, or even die, if they are simply labeled, drugged, and psychoanalyzed.

I've written *A Dose of Sanity* to show both patients and doctors that there is an alternative to DSM psychiatry, and that many "mental" disorders can be correctly diagnosed and effectively treated. I hope that psychiatrists who read this book will recognize it as constructive criticism, and that lay readers will be heartened by the message that there is hope for many people suffering from behavioral and emotional problems. Above all, I want readers to understand that *the brain is the organ of behavior,* and that all aberrant behavior stems from brain dysfunction. There is no "mind" without the brain—and there is no true psychiatric treatment that doesn't treat the brain.

I'd like to thank the many patients whose stories I've told in these pages. I owe them a debt of gratitude for allowing me to describe their suffering in an attempt to educate others.

I'd also like to acknowledge the efforts of Alison Blake, who has, through her enthusiasm, energy, intelligence, and ability to translate my "medical-ese" into English, made this book possible. I wish to acknowledge as well the perseverance of my agent, Margot Maley, and the outstanding vision of Kelly Franklin, my editor at Wiley, who realized that, bitter as the pill might be, the story of psychiatry's shortcomings has to be told. In addition, I am indebted to my office staff for assisting me with communications and rewrites and for allowing me to pursue this effort in concert with my other responsibilities. Finally, I wish to thank Chris Stave and the other librarians at UCSD Medical School for their efficiency and cheerful responsiveness to my requests.

SYDNEY WALKER III, M.D.

La Jolla, California
February 1996

Contents

CHAPTER I

Typhus, Tattoos, and Waterbeds

Missed Diagnoses and Cures that Kill

As long as diagnosis is in doubt, course and treatment are guesswork.

Melvin Gray, M.D.,
in *Neuroses: A Comprehensive and Critical View*

The mistaken assumption that the DSM is scientifically sound has led to confusion on the part of clinicians and to heartache on the part of patients and their families.

Therapist Paula Caplan,
in *They Say You're Crazy*

Typhus, tattoos, and waterbeds.
Faulty gas heaters, lead paint, and pinworms.
Brain tumors, eye drops, and pigeons.

WHAT DO ALL OF THESE HAVE IN COMMON? THEY'RE ALL potential causes of the strange, frightening, and debilitating symptoms that psychiatrists mistakenly label as "mental illness."

As a practicing psychiatrist and neurologist, I've successfully diagnosed and treated hundreds of patients whose emotional and behavioral symptoms were caused by tumors, infections, toxins, medication errors, genetic diseases, and other physical problems. Most of them came to me after being tagged with psychiatric labels—manic depression, anxiety disorder, attention deficit hyperactivity disorder—and being given powerful mind-altering drugs or referrals for psychotherapy. By the time they called my office,

1

many were desperate, some were suicidal, and few had been significantly helped. By the time they left my office, they *had* been helped—not because I'm any smarter than other psychiatrists, but because I've been well trained in the science of diagnosis.

Rachel's Story

One of these patients was Rachel Weiss, a tiny, silver-haired lady with apple cheeks and a concentration camp number tattooed on her arm.[1] Rachel was an American success story: a Holocaust survivor who came to the United States after World War II, became a successful musical artist, and married a wonderful man. At the time I examined her, however, she was a tormented and delusional woman.

Rachel had grown up in Holland, the well-loved child of an aging college professor and his violinist wife. A promising musician herself, Rachel began playing the piano at age five; later, as a teenager, she dreamed of touring the world as a concert pianist. But Rachel's childhood dreams ended when Adolf Hitler rose to power in Germany.

At age sixteen, Rachel—along with her mother and hundreds of other Jews in her community—was taken to a Nazi labor camp. There they were beaten routinely, raped by the prison guards, fed next to nothing, and forced to work sixteen-hour days. Rachel watched her mother die of starvation, and nearly died herself when dysentery and other infectious diseases swept through the camp. Liberated by the Americans, Rachel—reduced to a 70-pound skeleton—returned to her home, only to find that her father and most of her other relatives had been killed.

---

[1] Names and identifying details have been altered to protect patients' confidentiality.

The tragedies Rachel endured as a young girl would have destroyed many people, but she was a survivor. With a suitcase containing only a few items of clothing scrounged from a cousin, Rachel moved to New York to live with an aunt. She went to college, won a scholarship to a prestigious music academy, and landed a job with a local orchestra. A few years later, she married a talented cellist named Benjamin.

When I first saw Rachel, she was in her sixties, still happily married, and still a successful part-time musician. She did charity work for a local hospital and had mastered oil painting and gourmet cooking in her spare time. Although she continued to grieve for her lost family, and always would, she had come to terms with her tragic childhood and had survived it with great courage and grace. In short, she was a remarkably well-adjusted person—most of the time.

Several times a year, however, Rachel experienced terrifying "attacks." During an attack—like the one she was suffering when I examined her—she became, according to Benjamin, "someone I don't even recognize." Her symptoms included crippling bouts of fever, sweating, terrible despondency and hopelessness, and delusions. She wept, saw visions of her deceased parents, and became paranoid, accusing Benjamin of infidelity and treachery. She ranted that her fellow orchestra members were "out to get her." She imagined people stalking her, and thought her close friends were conspiring against her.

Dozens of psychiatrists had examined Rachel over the years. To them, her diagnosis was obvious: a severe depression caused by the horrors she had suffered in the Nazi labor camp, and by the deaths of her family members. Their prescriptions were obvious as well: years of psychotherapy, augmented by powerful antidepressant drugs. Unfortunately, neither of these approaches helped. Why not? Because the psychiatrists' diagnosis, no matter how "obvious," was wrong. Rachel *had* suffered terribly, and indeed bore deep emotional scars. But the culprit that was directly to blame for her cyclical attacks of paranoia and despondency was not the Nazis, but typhus.

During World War II, typhus ran rampant in most concentration camps, killing thousands and infecting thousands more who survived. Many of the survivors now suffer from a well-known syndrome known as "recrudescent rickettsial infection," or Brill-Zinsser disease. The agent that causes the disorder, *Rickettsia prowazekii,* is transmitted to humans by lice. It can infect a human, lie dormant for decades, and then resurface to cause fever, rash, headache, and emotional symptoms including paranoia, despondency, and hopelessness. Doctors can treat the disease easily with common antibiotics—but only if they're alert enough to recognize it. Unfortunately, many Nazi prison camp survivors with Brill-Zinsser disease don't get antibiotics; instead, like Rachel, they get antidepressants and years of expensive psychotherapy.

Fortunately, Rachel's story had a happy ending: I discovered that her bizarre symptoms were, indeed, caused by the typhus that had infected her decades earlier. Rachel was enormously relieved to learn that her condition wasn't "mental illness" but rather a treatable infection, and that the antibiotic therapy for the disease that had crippled her for decades was so simple that she didn't even need to be hospitalized for treatment. She was also relieved to learn that she no longer needed to take toxic drugs or undergo hours of psychotherapy—the only two treatments she'd received during all the years she'd suffered.

An Epidemic of Nondiagnosis

Literally thousands of Americans, like Rachel, are suffering from undiagnosed and untreated brain disorders. These patients are victims of a dangerous trend in modern psychiatry: the *failure to diagnose.* The "depressed" patient with Brill-Zinsser disease, the "hyperactive" child who actually suffers from chronic low-level carbon monoxide poisoning, the "anxious" housewife with a thyroid disorder, and the "conduct-disordered" teenager with subclinical beriberi all can be cured—but not if their doctors fail to diagnose what's really wrong with them.

Such patients eventually learn the hard way that *a label is not a diagnosis.* Saying someone is "depressed" or "anxious" is a far cry from finding out what causes the depression or anxiety; it's comparable to a pediatrician saying a child has "spots," without bothering to find out whether the spots are caused by measles, poison ivy, or staphylococcus. Patients who have been "diagnosed" as having manic depression, anxiety disorder, attention deficit hyperactivity disorder, and so on, *haven't been diagnosed;* they've merely been described. Such labels, as psychiatrist Matthew P. Dumont has noted, are simply a sophisticated-sounding way of making quick and superficial observations.

Robert L. Taylor, a physician and the author of *Mind or Body,* points out that terms such as anxious, depressed, paranoid, catatonic, and manic "signify nothing with respect to specific causation," and notes that *"descriptive labeling does not provide causative understanding"* (italics in original). And causative understanding—knowing why symptoms occur—is the foundation of medical care.

Doctors are trained to begin with a patient's symptoms, and work from there—by taking compulsively thorough medical and personal histories, conducting in-depth physical and neurological examinations, ordering appropriate neurophysiological evaluations and biochemical studies, and evaluating the results of brain scans and other tests, until a definitive diagnosis can be made. This medical detective work, known as the *deductive differential diagnosis,* is the cornerstone of medicine. But modern psychiatry has attempted to shortcut the process with a book known as the *Diagnostic and Statistical Manual* (DSM, currently in its fourth revision). In doing so, psychiatry has replaced the science of diagnosis with the pseudoscience of labeling.

DSM, the professional bible of American psychiatrists, is published by the American Psychiatric Association (APA). It is, quite simply, a catalog of symptoms—for instance, "has hallucinations," "is aloof," "has difficulty sleeping." If a patient has enough of the symptoms listed in any cluster, he or she can be "diagnosed" straight from the book—without benefit of lab tests, brain scans, a physical exam, or the taking of a careful medical history.

For example, using DSM, a person can be "diagnosed" as having "attention deficit/hyperactivity disorder" simply on the basis that he or she exhibits six or more of the following symptoms for at least six months, to a degree that is "maladaptive" and impairs functioning:

1. Often fidgets with hands or feet or squirms in seat.
2. Often leaves seat in classroom or in other situations in which remaining seated is expected.
3. Often runs about or climbs excessively in situations in which it is inappropriate (in adolescents or adults, may be limited to subjective feelings of restlessness).
4. Often has difficulty playing or engaging in leisure activities quietly.
5. Is often "on the go" or often acts as if "driven by a motor."
6. Often talks excessively.
7. Often blurts out answers before questions have been completed.
8. Often has difficulty awaiting turn.
9. Often interrupts or intrudes on others (e.g., butts into conversations or games).

Using DSM, a person can be "diagnosed" as having "anxiety disorder," if significant worry or anxiety is associated with three or more of the following symptoms:

1. Restlessness.
2. Fatigue.
3. Difficulty concentrating.
4. Irritability.
5. Muscle tension.
6. Sleep disturbance.

In short, with DSM, the psychiatrist no longer needs to spend tedious hours searching for the reasons *why* a patient suffers from fatigue, anxiety, dizziness, or other symptoms. He or she simply has to identify a sufficient number of such symptoms to shoehorn the patient into a "diagnostic" category.

The authors of DSM-IV and its counterpart, ICD-10 (the latest version of the International Classification of Diseases, published by the World Health Organization and used by European psychiatrists) warn against using the manuals as medical "cookbooks"—add enough symptomatic ingredients and you have a diagnosis—but it's standard practice to use them in precisely this way. Although DSM-IV's authors stress that "the specific diagnostic criteria included in DSM-IV are meant to serve as guidelines to be informed by clinical judgment," psychiatrists too often use DSM as a substitute for—not an adjunct to—differential diagnosis.

The overreliance on DSM is not solely the fault of individual psychiatrists; to a large degree, they are victims of a system built entirely on the myth of the DSM "diagnosis." In the four decades since it was first published (in 1952), DSM has gradually become the established diagnostic language of the psychiatric community: hospitals expect psychiatric patients' medical records to list DSM labels, psychiatric journals almost exclusively publish articles using accepted DSM terms, and insurance companies now require that individuals seeking reimbursement for psychiatric treatment submit the DSM names and codes of their disorders. (Psychology researcher Robyn Dawes comments, in *House of Cards,* "I know several people whose psychiatrists or psychologists have actually apologized for their official diagnosis: 'I have to label you this way in order to be reimbursed. Please don't pay too much attention to the label.' Imagine a medical doctor apologizing for labeling an ulcer an ulcer, explaining that the label is a matter of convenience for being reimbursed!") Even patients know the DSM lingo, and often are disappointed if they leave a psychiatrist's office without a DSM label and a prescription for Prozac. DSM is popular because it works for the system: drug companies, insurers, and hospitals. A psychiatrist who bucks the DSM trend often suffers, both financially and professionally.

Unfortunately, there's a big catch to the DSM "diagnostic" method: the impressive medical terms in the DSM conceal a myriad of underlying medical problems, many of them curable—and many of them dangerous if left untreated. Most of these problems are surprisingly easy to uncover, using standard medical tests, careful questioning, and good deductive reasoning. For instance, I've successfully treated "hyperactive" children whose problems were caused by lead or carbon monoxide poisoning, anemia, low glucose levels, poor calcium intake, brain lesions, parasites—even tight underwear! Had these children received a standard "diagnosis" of attention deficit hyperactivity disorder, most would be taking Ritalin for decades—and many would still be crippled by symptoms of hyperactivity.

Here's an example of how a DSM cookbook diagnosis can overlook a serious, and readily treatable, physical problem causing classic symptoms of hyperactivity.

Frankie, a frail, peaked eleven-year-old boy, came to my office recently with his distraught parents, who were at their wits' end because of his aggression and uncontrolled tantrums. Frankie couldn't pay attention at school, was falling behind in his classes, and had lost many of his friends because of his difficult behavior. The week before, he'd been suspended for throwing punches at a classmate, and he was always in trouble either for daydreaming or for fighting. When I questioned him gently about school and hobbies, he was sullen and defensive—obviously believing I was yet another grown-up who wanted to know why he was always "bad."

Frankie had more than enough symptoms to qualify for a label of attention deficit hyperactivity disorder, according to DSM-IV. I could have written him a prescription for Ritalin and sent the family on their way, and many psychiatrists would have said I'd done my job. The parents would have been grateful too, because Ritalin—although it wouldn't have cured their child—might have at least reduced his trying behavior problems.

But "diagnosis" means finding the *cause* of a disorder, not just giving it a name. In Frankie's case, the first clues that led me to a diagnosis were his unhealthy appearance and the blue veins that stood out on the sides of his head. More clues came from questioning Frankie and his parents. He told me that he fought with the other kids because he was angry about "always being the last kid picked for baseball." He was also the last kid picked for basketball, for tag, and for soccer. Why? "I can't play for very long before I get worn out," he explained. His parents told me that Frankie was always tired, even when he first got up in the morning—a common symptom of cardiac disorders.

My initial suspicions were that Frankie's "behavioral" problem was actually a heart problem, and that his aggression was a natural result of his frustration at not being able to keep up. My suspicions grew when my physical examination revealed ridged nails, cyanotic (bluish) skin color, and other signs of cardiac disease. Extensive tests uncovered the root of Frankie's problems: he suffered from a heart defect that reduced oxygenation of his blood, and his brain was literally starving for oxygen. The problem was corrected, and Frankie's behavior and school performance began to improve. (Last I heard, he'd also found out he was pretty good at football.) Frankie's recovery was due not to a temporary panacea like Ritalin, but to an informed evaluation that uncovered the real reason for his disorder.

Then there was Linda, a small, freckle-faced seven-year-old I evaluated years ago. Linda, whose parents had died in a car accident, was living in a facility for children awaiting adoption. Described as a "pest" who was cranky and jittery in class, she was very bright but classified as "unmotivated." She had trouble falling asleep, slept badly, and awoke grumpy and tired. She'd taken Ritalin for a year, even though it had little beneficial effect (and caused side effects, including a facial tic), and might have taken similar drugs for decades if a bright social worker hadn't brought her in for another opinion.

Indeed, I did have another opinion—which was that Linda's other doctors hadn't tried very hard to diagnose her. One look at Linda should have given any careful physician a good idea of what ailed her. While she wasn't filthy, she wasn't very clean, either. Her fingernails had a crust of dirt under them, her hair was unkempt, and her ankles could have used a good scrubbing. A quick glance at her clothes confirmed that she hadn't changed her underwear in a couple of days.

It didn't take me long to determine that Linda suffered from pinworms, a relatively minor but very irritating parasitic infection that affects as many as one-fifth of children in the United States at any given time. Pinworms, while common everywhere, are often epidemic in group settings, such as Linda's adoption agency, where large numbers of children with less than adequate hygiene live and play closely together. Pinworms lay their eggs in the anal area, causing itching and tickling which are particularly bothersome at night. Poor Linda wasn't suffering from hyperactivity, but from chronic fatigue—the result of years of sleeplessness due to itching. I prescribed treatment for her—and recommended that all of the children at her residential facility be checked and treated for pinworms as well.

Like Linda and Frankie, thousands of "hyperactive" children are taking Ritalin for toxic, infectious, metabolic, or neurodegenerative disorders. But Ritalin won't treat these disorders; all it will do is help conceal the fact that they *haven't been treated*, by masking symptoms crying out for a diagnosis.

For patients labeled as "psychotic," the risks of improper diagnosis (or rather, nondiagnosis) are higher still. Thousands of patients suffer serious side effects from potent psychiatric medications, many become addicted, and more than a few die of aplastic anemia and other drug-induced disorders. Some commit suicide, driven to despair by their failure to find relief. The tragedy is that many of them could have been diagnosed and treated successfully without ever resorting to psychiatric drugs or psychotherapy (a treatment that can help patients deal with the emotional consequences of brain dysfunction, but is *not* a replacement for medical diagnosis and treatment of biological disorders). Here are some examples of near-tragedies, from my case files.

Antonio, a handsome, soft-spoken, 40-year-old businessman with an elegantly styled pompadour of brown hair, came to me suffering from despondency, fatigue, and anxiety. "I've run my own company for decades," he told me, "but now I hardly have the energy to get out of bed and go into the office. I feel like I'm trying to move underwater—everything is so hard." In addition, Antonio said he suffered from dizzy spells and a bothersome ringing in his ears that kept him awake at night. I could have given Antonio a DSM label of depression, a prescription for antidepressants, and a referral to a psychotherapist. If I had, I would have endangered not only his life but the lives of his wife and his mistress as well.

While taking an extensive medical and personal history, I learned that, in his younger days, Antonio had served in Vietnam. During furlough trips to Japan, he'd gotten many tattoos which he'd later had removed. To any good doctor, the word "tattoo" immediately raises suspicions of syphilis, which is frequently transmitted by dirty tattoo needles. Syphilis, called the "great imitator," mimics symptoms of many psychiatric disorders. The symptoms often appear "out of nowhere," after a latent period of years or even decades.

A laboratory study called an FTA-Abs, and follow-up tests, confirmed that Antonio had seronegative syphilis (a form that can be contracted from contaminated tattoo needles and is not detectable by standard blood tests such as premarital screenings). I treated him with penicillin and his symptoms disappeared.

If Antonio had been given a DSM "diagnosis" of depression and a prescription for Prozac, he might have felt better for a little while, under the influence of the drug. But he wouldn't have felt good for very long, because Prozac won't cure syphilis. And prescribing Prozac for Antonio wouldn't have helped his wife or his girlfriend, both of whom also tested positive for syphilis.

Jane, another of my patients, was a svelte, 66-year-old widow who looked twenty years younger than her real age—a definite advantage in her career as a flamboyant cabaret singer. But Jane's career hit the rocks when she abruptly developed anxiety, stomachaches, sweating, ringing in her ears, and dizziness. She also began sleeping badly, and she awoke exhausted every morning. Formerly an active and vivacious woman fond of parties and late nights on the town, Jane had spent the past year at home taking powerful antianxiety drugs. She'd stopped dating, canceled all of her performances, and shut herself off from family and friends. "I used to feel like I was sixty going on twenty," she told me. "Now I feel like sixty going on ninety."

Jane had been admitted to a psychiatric hospital and had even contemplated committing suicide. Her DSM label: classic panic disorder. The recommended treatments: Xanax and psychotherapy. But the drug, the psychotherapy, and the hospitalization didn't help Jane a bit. That's because Jane didn't have "panic disorder"; she had a serious medical problem that wasn't being treated.

A careful examination and history revealed that Jane's symptoms began shortly after she reduced her dose of thyroid medication, which she'd taken for many years for a condition known as hypothyroidism (underactivity of the thyroid gland). Hypothyroidism causes the heart, intestines, and other organs to "slow down," leading to symptoms such as cold feet, weight gain, dry and lifeless hair, dry skin, a deep voice, hearing loss, and heavy menstrual periods. Hypothyroidism also can cause drastic changes in personality and behavior. The patient often feels "achy," and even simple tasks like preparing a meal become overwhelming. Many patients lose all interest in sex. Some, like Jane, become suicidally despondent or anxious.

I put Jane back on her thyroid medication, and her symptoms began to disappear almost immediately. In the meantime, I'd also discovered that Jane had inner-ear problems that were causing her dizziness. I prescribed a medication to handle her inner-ear disorder (which was also alleviated by treatment of her thyroid disorder), and told her to replace her waterbed with a regular mattress because waterbeds often contribute to sleep disturbance in individuals with inner-ear problems. Jane was back to normal— and back to singing—in a matter of weeks.

The moral is that *very little is undiagnosable, but much is not being diagnosed*. Psychiatrists who fail to find the real causes of mental disorders (or, more correctly, brain dysfunctions) cannot possibly treat them effectively. Indeed, the drug "treatments" commonly prescribed after tagging a patient with a DSM label often don't treat at all; they merely mask symptoms. And although drugs often provide temporary relief, they always do so at a price. The patient on Halcion who commits suicide, the child on Ritalin who feels like a zombie, and the anxious patient who becomes addicted to Valium, all have suffered unnecessarily, if their symptoms were caused by treatable physical disorders. Patients who spend years undergoing psychoanalysis based on DSM labels are victims too, if they have physical problems that could have been accurately diagnosed and cured.

Cases like these are not, as psychiatrists would like to think, isolated incidents. In 1982, Robert Hoffman reported that, of 215 patients admitted to a medical-psychiatric hospital unit, 41 percent were initially misdiagnosed; in addition, he found that 63 percent of patients labeled as having "untreatable dementia" actually had treatable disorders. M. M. Herring, in a 1985 study of 131 randomly selected patients at the Manhattan Psychiatric Center, found that "approximately 75 percent of the patients reevaluated may have been wrongly diagnosed when admitted to the center," and that "frequent misdiagnosis of schizophrenia caused severe harm to many patients who were inappropriately given powerful drugs, such as neuroleptics [drugs affecting the nervous system], that mask symptoms and may cause irreversible side effects." Erwin Koranyi's studies in the 1980s found that psychiatrists misdiagnosed about half of patients with detectable physical illnesses; commenting that "psychiatrists often lose their skills of performing competent physical examination," Koranyi cited a survey in which *none* of 100 psychiatrists questioned said that they performed routine physical examinations on their patients.

More recent research reveals that, even with modern laboratory and brain imaging technologies available to them, psychiatrists often fail to diagnose obvious physical problems in their patients. In 1990, Lorrin Koran and colleagues, who examined 529 randomly selected patients in eight treatment programs in a state mental health system, found that nearly 38 percent of those patients had a significant, detectable physical disease—but less than half of them had been diagnosed. The harm done by such misdiagnosis and nondiagnosis can last forever. As Koran points out, "A physical disease incorrectly diagnosed as a mental disease can lead to a lifetime on psychotropic drugs, loss of productivity, physical and social deterioration and shattered dreams."

"People with real or alleged psychiatric or behavioral disorders are being misdiagnosed—and harmed—to an astonishing degree," Charles B. Inlander, president of The People's Medical Society, and his colleagues say in *Medicine on Trial*. "Many of them do not have psychiatric problems but exhibit physical symptoms that may mimic mental conditions, and so they are misdiagnosed, put on drugs, put in institutions, and sent into a limbo from which they may never return. . . . On the other hand, the physical illnesses of psychiatric patients go underdiagnosed or undiagnosed." Famed neurologist Sir Francis Walshe has charged that mental hospitals "are living museums of undiscovered bodily disease . . . undiagnosed but not undiagnosable."

An accurate diagnosis doesn't always mean a cure. Diagnosing a psychiatric patient as having a brain tumor, or multiple sclerosis, or lupus, doesn't mean I can always help the patient. (Any patient is better off with an accurate diagnosis, however, because there's always a chance, given the rapid rate of medical discoveries, that a treatment or cure will become available.) And there are occasions when it's impossible—even with state-of-the-art technology and careful differential diagnosis—to determine the cause of a patient's symptoms. In such a case, however, I'm able to *rule out* hundreds of possible causes and to establish a baseline that may later help me detect the emergence of telltale signs of a diagnosable disorder. I'm also able to avoid potentially dangerous treatments for disorders the patient doesn't have. (This is much more important than it sounds. A remarkable number of patients today suffer from "iatrogenic"—literally, "doctor-caused"—disorders traceable to unnecessary and harmful medications or surgeries.)

But in a surprisingly large percentage of cases labeled as "mental" disorders, there *is* a diagnosable physical problem, and that problem *does* have a treatment or even a cure.

Why Patients Buy Into the DSM Myth

DSM labels don't cure. Neither do psychotropic drugs and psychotherapy, the two treatments that almost always follow a DSM "diagnosis." Powerful drugs such as Thorazine, Valium, and Xanax often cause as many symptoms as they alleviate. And psychotherapy may help a patient cope with disturbing symptoms, but it won't cure an underlying brain dysfunction. In short, simply naming a patient's symptoms doesn't help a psychiatrist understand or correct these symptoms.

Bear in mind that a label is simply a name—much like the names of your friends. And, to quote Mr. Shakespeare, "What's in a name?" Everything—and nothing. Calling your friends "Sam" and "Bertha" and "Susan" helps you to get their attention, or to describe them to others, but it doesn't tell you anything about what makes them tick. Similarly, labeling patients as "depressed" or "anxious" may allow a psychiatrist to group them conveniently, but it won't reveal anything about the causes of their problems. A psychiatrist who believes that all "depressed" patients are alike is as misguided as a person who believes that all people named "Jim" are alike. Both labels are handy, but neither is very informative.

In other words, a patient with syphilis, or a brain tumor, or a thyroid disorder, isn't any better off after being labeled as "depressed" or "anxious" than before receiving the label from the psychiatrist. Since that's the case, why don't patients complain about receiving DSM labels instead of diagnoses?

For one thing, DSM labels reassure patients. The symptoms of brain dysfunction often are terribly frightening. Patients worry that they are "going crazy," and that they are losing their basic humanity. They may suffer for months before seeing a doctor. Just hearing from the psychiatrist that their symptoms have a name is tremendously comforting—especially when the psychiatrist also offers a "magic pill" as treatment.

Psychiatrist E. Fuller Torrey, who has compared psychiatrists and native witch doctors, says that both groups rely heavily on the "magic" of naming. The very act of naming a disorder has a therapeutic effect, Torrey says, whether it involves a psychiatrist "diagnosing" depression or a witch doctor "diagnosing" possession by evil spirits. "Every therapist who has ever had the experience of observing a patient's relief after solemnly telling him that he was suffering from idiopathic dermatitis or pediculosis knows how important the name is," Torrey notes in *The Mind Game: Witchdoctors and Psychiatrists*. "It says to the patient that someone understands, that he is not alone with his sickness, and implicitly that there is a way to get well. It is used by all therapists everywhere, witch doctors and psychiatrists equally effectively." Torrey cites the observations of psychiatrist G. M. Carstairs, who had watched a healer in rural India:

> What was expected from the healer was reassurance. So long as the illness was nameless, patients felt desperately afraid, but once its magic origin had been defined and the appropriate measures taken, they could face the outcome calmly. The parallel with our own clinical experience is obvious.

The authors of the latest DSM acknowledge the power of simply naming a disorder. "Patients often feel uniquely damned—like they're the first person to invent a particular problem," DSM-IV chairman Allen Frances recently commented. "But the DSM shows them their problems are generally so common and well-described that they're right down there on paper. This can be very relieving."

Psychiatric patients frequently *do* feel a little better after receiving a DSM label, simply because brain symptoms are exacerbated by the biochemistry of stress—and there is little in life more stressful than worrying about going insane. Many patients experience a phenomenon known as the "flight into health" when they learn (1) that their disorder has a name, and (2) that it isn't fatal. The flight into health is a natural uplifting of the spirits, which may make a patient feel, erroneously, that his or her condition is clearing up. And because most patients initially respond to psychotropic medications, they generally do appear—at least for a while—to be getting better.

But "depressed" patients who actually suffer from brain tumors, toxic exposure, hormonal imbalances, colitis, postinfectious disorders, anemia, or autoimmune diseases *aren't cured* when a psychiatrist tells them they're "depressed," and they aren't cured by taking Xanax, Valium, or Prozac. They are cured only if the brain dysfunctions causing their disorders are diagnosed and corrected.

What's Happened to Diagnosis?

Psychiatrists are doctors. They all go to medical school, just like gynecologists or cardiologists. While they're in medical school, they learn to examine patients, develop strategies for evaluation, and make diagnoses. They also learn that "mental" disorders can be caused by brain tumors, viruses, metabolic defects, and hundreds of other physical disorders. Furthermore, like other doctors, psychiatrists are dedicated professionals who want to do their best for their patients. Why, when they go into practice, do so many of them fail to use all of their training?

One reason is that many doctors choose psychiatry because, after entering the field of medicine, they find out that they don't particularly care for it. Some doctors have difficulty mastering the art of examining patients, don't like touching people (particularly people with unpleasant or contagious diseases), or feel inadequate when confronted with the tremendous amount of diagnostic "grunt work" required to be a good gynecologist, neurologist, or urologist. Psychiatrist Jerrold Maxmen quotes one of his colleagues as saying: "The sights and feel of medicine were all wrong for me. I hated sticking people to draw blood or putting in IVs; all that poking around . . . I don't like touching sick people." The visceral dislike of medicine among many psychiatrists is a primary reason why DSM is popular (after all, you don't need to touch a patient to administer a DSM label) and hands-on diagnosis is not.

Another reason is human nature: we tend to assume that "if everyone else is doing it, it must be right," and virtually everyone in psychiatry is currently using DSM as a definitive diagnostic manual. Most of a psychiatrist's specialty training, in fact, centers around learning how to make accurate DSM "diagnoses," which drugs to prescribe for each DSM label, and which forms of psychotherapy to recommend for each DSM category. This misguided instruction is the fault of the American Psychiatric Association (APA), which publishes DSM and sets the standards for psychiatric training, and not necessarily the fault of individual psychiatrists—who are, for the most part, simply doing what they've been taught.

The field of psychiatry is so dependent on DSM that it has spawned an entire industry. The American Psychiatric Press (the publishing arm of the APA) publishes not only DSM but half a dozen spin-off products that, combined with DSM, grossed the APA over *$22 million* in 1993 alone. Although many psychiatrists' offices lack even rudimentary medical diagnostic equipment, virtually all have at least one copy of DSM. Because almost all practitioners, from the board of the American Psychiatric Association on down, are using DSM "diagnoses" and consider them valid, the average psychiatrist no doubt assumes that he or she is practicing state-of-the-art medicine when using DSM-IV.

The average psychiatrist may also assume that DSM accurately reflects the consensus of the medical community, and that DSM is supported by careful scientific research. However, nothing could be further from the truth. In reality, the labels that appear in DSM are voted on by panels of psychiatrists who spend years fighting over them—and the final decisions these dueling parties make are based on politics far more often than on medical knowledge.

Take "self-defeating personality disorder," for instance. Male and female psychiatrists working on DSM-III-R (the "R" stands for "Revised") in the late 1980s fought bitterly for over a year about whether to include this term, which is used to describe self-sacrificing people (usually women) who choose careers or relationships that are likely to cause disappointment. Female psychiatrists dubbed this label the "good-wife syndrome," saying that the term made the behavior of normal females—who generally are more willing than men to put others' needs before theirs—sound pathological. (Several female psychiatrists went further and called it "psychiatrist's wife syndrome," pointing out that a large number of psychiatrists' wives sacrifice their own education to help put their husbands through medical school—after which their husbands are likely to divorce them for younger women!) The American Psychological Association (whose members also use the DSM extensively) was so angered at the proposed category that it urged its members to boycott its use. And therapist Paula Caplan, noting that there was no similar label for typical male behaviors—domination, poor communication skills, preoccupation with sex, and so on—suggested, only somewhat tongue-in-cheek, that the DSM authors consider adding a label of "delusional dominating personality disorder." Caplan's suggestion was dismissed rather huffily by DSM's largely male authors, but "self-defeating personality disorder" was voted in as a "provisional" label—only to be voted out in the next DSM.

Then there was the Great PMS Debate. Many psychiatrists working on DSM-III-R wanted premenstrual syndrome (PMS) included as a "diagnosis." Many others charged that this would designate hundreds of thousands of women in America as mentally disordered. After almost coming to blows, the DSM authors decided to include PMS in the manual's appendix (a dumping ground for categories "needing further study") under the label of "late luteal phase dysphoric disorder." Continuing dissatisfaction with this label led the authors of DSM-IV to change the name to "premenstrual dysphoric disorder," although no one seems sure why this would make it less controversial. Displeasure with the category continues, yet premenstrual dysphoric disorder—although still consigned to the back of the DSM—has an official code number, implying that it is an agreed-on "diagnosis."

The controversies over PMS and self-defeating personality disorder pale, however, in comparison to the debate over homosexuality as a "diagnosis." This battle first took shape in the 1970s, when gay activists (including members of the Gay Psychiatric Association) began picketing APA conferences to protest the designation of homosexuality as a disorder in DSM-II. Psychoanalysts, who had a considerable stake in retaining this "diagnosis," retaliated by threatening mutiny if the designation were changed. Years of protests and debates led to a ballot in which the entire membership of the APA was literally asked to vote for or against the concept of homosexuality as a disorder. The upshot is that homosexuality—a "disorder" in DSM-II—is considered a normal condition in later DSMs. Yet, childhood "gender identity disorder"—the strongest single predictor of homosexuality—is still listed as an abnormal condition. Confused? You're not alone.

"To read about the evolution of the DSM," Louise Armstrong says in *And They Call It Help*, "is to know this: It is an entirely political document. What it includes, what it does not include, are the result of intensive campaigning, lengthy negotiating, infighting, and power plays."

An excellent example of the politics and the nonscience—or nonsense—behind DSM is the story of "self-defeating personality disorder." As I mentioned, it was included in DSM-III-R, only to be excluded in DSM-IV. But how did "self-defeating personality disorder" become a "diagnosis" in the first place? Not because there was any demand for it; in fact, there was outrage from many psychiatrists who believed the label could be used to blame women for abuse by their spouses. Furthermore, there wasn't any research base to support the validity of the term. According to several participants in the DSM deliberations, the real reason "self-defeating personality disorder" was included in DSM-III-R was that three psychiatrists (including Robert Spitzer, the chairman of the DSM-III-R committee) thought up the label while on a fishing trip. When they returned from the trip, they persuaded colleagues at their medical center to conduct one study on the new "disorder," presented it to the DSM-III-R committee, and— *voila!*—an entirely new mental illness was born.

DSM's authors claim that the manual's validity is supported by field trials involving hundreds of clinicians and patients, but these trials simply gauge how well clinicians can be trained to apply each label to patients—without regard to whether the labels are accurate. (As Paula Caplan has pointed out, "One could get a large group of people to agree to call all horses 'unicorns' . . . but that would not mean that any of them ever really saw unicorns.") Even in this limited sense, DSM is a failure because the ability of psychiatrists to agree on patients' labels—that is, their "interrater reliability"—has proven to be very poor. And, according to an in-depth analysis by university professors Stuart Kirk and Herb Kutchins, the field trials the authors of DSM brag about are so poorly designed that they are close to meaningless.

The result, inevitably, is that the final terms published in various editions of DSM reflect panel members' personal biases and beliefs rather than any valid research. Attorney Jean Matulis, a critic of DSM's pervasive influence not only on psychiatry but on legal proceedings as well, has called it "the collective hunches of a bunch of people." Paula Caplan, who recently argued with the DSM panel over several labels, commented angrily afterward that the committee's deliberations were rife with "pseudoscience and sloppy science," adding that "there is a breathtaking arrogance about those people that allows them to say things they can't begin to support." Renee Garfinkel, who attended DSM-III-R meetings on behalf of the American Psychological Association, agrees; she told *Time* magazine that "the low level of intellectual effort was shocking. Diagnoses were developed by majority vote on the level we would use to choose a restaurant. . . . It may reflect on our naïveté, but it was our belief that there would be an attempt to look at things scientifically."

The nonscientific approach used to create DSM leads to irrational and constantly changing diagnostic criteria: a patient might be perfectly normal according to one version of DSM and mentally ill by the standards of the next. (For instance, "narcissistic personality disorder"—used to describe vain people who are self-centered and frequently take advantage of others—was a DSM "diagnosis" until 1968. It was eliminated from the version used between 1968 and 1980, but was reinstated in 1980. Thus, a self-centered, vain person was "mentally ill" before 1968, normal for the next twelve years, and then "mentally ill" again after 1980.) And a "diagnosis" might be based on the silliest of rationales; for instance, former psychoanalyst Jeffrey Moussaieff Masson notes in *Final Analysis* that, under DSM-III-R, "for a patient to state that a therapist [was] boring or uninteresting [was] a primary sign of what is now called 'the self-defeating personality disorder.'"

Such arbitrary labels are not just silly; they are dangerous to a patient's health, career, and personal life. Once a DSM label is on a patient's chart, it stays there for life—and the consequences can be devastating. A DSM label of "depression," for instance, can make it virtually impossible for a patient to obtain private health insurance, even if the patient has recovered from his or her symptoms. The label can weigh heavily against a parent in a custody battle. It can also scare off potential employers. As Caplan says, "One cannot stress enough the havoc wrought in people's lives when they are given labels that are unwarranted and unhelpful."

It's frightening that lives can be ruined by DSM labels based not on scientific consensus but, as one critic has said, on "chummy, anecdotal reports of one believer to another." It's appalling that labels affecting millions of Americans—and possibly costing them their jobs, their children, or their reputations—are determined by political intrigue and personal bias. But even if every psychiatrist in the country agreed on every DSM term, and the committees that developed DSM were totally apolitical, DSM would still be frightening because it ignores the causes of the symptoms it labels.

DSM and the Decline of Psychiatry

DSM, in a way, reflects the history of psychiatry itself. The first psychiatrists were excellent diagnosticians who were convinced that most mental symptoms could be traced to bodily disease. Wilhelm Griesinger, in the 1800s, believed that insanity involved changes in the brain's anatomy. So did one of the first true giants in the field of psychiatry, the German doctor Emil Kraepelin. (Kraepelin's textbooks were, in many respects, forerunners of the DSM—except that, *after* describing and categorizing his patients' symptoms, Kraepelin included thoughtful discussions of the possible physical causes of these symptoms.) Kraepelin surrounded himself with like-minded psychiatrists, including Alzheimer (who identified the disease named after him), Nissl (who developed a staining technique that allows researchers to see brain cells clearly under a microscope), and Brodmann (who discovered that different areas of the brain have different functions and contain different types of cells). All were dedicated to discovering the underlying physical causes of brain disorders—even though little or no technology for studying the brain existed at the time.

American psychiatry originally had strong biological underpinnings. Benjamin Rush (1746–1813), considered the father of American psychiatry, was noted for his insistence that insanity is a disease. A heroic doctor who joined the Continental Army as a surgeon (after making history as a signer of the Declaration of Independence), Rush was highly trained not only in psychiatry but in obstetrics, pediatrics, geriatrics, and the treatment of tuberculosis.

His *Diseases of the Mind,* written in 1812, was a landmark treatise on mental illness.

Biologically oriented psychiatry, heavily based on scientific research and documentation, prevailed into the early 1940s under the influence of the late Dr. Adolph Meyer, a professor of psychiatry at Johns Hopkins. There are stories of Dr. Meyer spending hours in his laboratory looking at brain slices, trying to find specific lesions that caused behavioral abnormalities. Meyer, with his emphasis on causation, insisted that psychiatric labels include the phrase "in reaction to," in recognition of the fact that "mental" disorders represent reactions to biological factors. But Meyer's influence faded toward the end of his career, and those who followed—including Walter Barton, Henry Work, George Tarjan, and Robert Pasnau—shifted psychiatry's focus from logic to labeling. By the time DSM-II was published in 1968, the phrase "in reaction to" was gone, and the label itself was considered a sufficient "diagnosis." Thus, the precise science of diagnosis gave way to the imprecise and inaccurate pseudoscience of labeling—a change that altered the course of psychiatry and, in effect, removed it from the field of medicine.

This change was facilitated in large part by the ascendancy, in the 1940s and 1950s, of psychoanalytically oriented Freudian and post-Freudian psychiatrists whose primary interest was in "the mind"—as though the mind could be considered as totally unrelated to the brain. By the 1950s, the brain was largely ignored by the very profession that specialized in understanding its output. In fact, most of the psychiatric therapies developed during the mid-1900s, which influenced DSM-I and later editions of this "diagnostic" manual, weren't even developed by medical doctors. Bruno Bettelheim, Carl Rogers, Anna Freud, Erich Fromm, and Erik Erikson were all psychologists, with little or no formal training in medicine or science. "Such a degree of nonmedical participation is totally inconceivable in surgery, obstetrics, or any other of the true medical specialties," psychiatrist E. Fuller Torrey notes. But then, psychiatrists in the psychoanalytic era weren't concerned with body tissues, hormones, bones, blood, or anything else that normal doctors treated; instead, they were dealing with an intangible, invisible "psyche." Although these psychiatrists conceded that a few disorders—pellagra, syphilis, stroke—could cause brain dysfunction leading to mental symptoms, most of them firmly believed that these were the exception rather than the rule. Instead, they attributed schizophrenia, depression, anxiety, autism, and a host of other psychoses and neuroses to psychic trauma caused by adverse events, particularly during childhood. Psychiatrists convinced that psychoses and neuroses stemmed from Oedipal complexes, ego dystonia, or authoritarian parenting had little interest in investigating brain dysfunction; thus, simplistic labels such as "depressed" or "masochistic" or "melancholic" were more than adequate for their purposes.

In recent decades, however, it has become clear that the promises of psychoanalysis were empty. The growing realization that psychoses and many more minor "mental" disorders are biologically caused has greatly reduced the ranks of psychoanalytic psychiatrists, and claims that psychotherapy can cure serious mental illness have been largely abandoned. Major changes in medicine—including advances in gene mapping and brain imaging technology—have encouraged psychiatry to move back toward its biological roots.

Unfortunately, it hasn't moved far enough to regain its position as a true medical science. Although psychiatry claims to have entered a scientific era, it still clings to a DSM system based on labeling rather than on diagnosis, and on guesswork and subjective interpretation rather than on diagnostic skills and scientific research. And psychiatry still fails, far too often, to attribute disturbances of thought and emotion to the brain—the very organ of thought and emotion. Both DSM's authors and psychiatry itself have forgotten the dictum of Adolph Meyer: symptoms of behavioral disorders occur *in reaction to* brain dysfunction, and a DSM label does nothing to identify such dysfunction, and even less to remediate it.

Does DSM Have a Future?

DSM labels may be useful for marriage counselors, social workers, teachers, and other nonmedical professionals whose goal is not to diagnose and cure, but to comfort and aid. But psychiatrists are medical doctors—and it's a doctor's job to diagnose diseases, not just to label them.

There is increasing evidence that psychiatrists realize this, and are dissatisfied with the elevation of DSM to a diagnostic religion. In a 1986 survey, for instance, nearly half of the psychiatrists polled doubted the validity of DSM-III "diagnostic" criteria, and 35 percent said they would stop using it if it weren't required. And DSM-IV, far from being accepted unquestioningly, was the subject of much acrimonious debate in the psychiatric community.

Psychiatrists are becoming increasingly aware that their field hasn't kept up with modern science, and many are calling for higher scientific standards in psychiatry. There is a growing discontent among psychiatrists regarding the poor quality of psychiatric "diagnosis" and research over the past few decades, as well as a growing realization that advances made in other medical fields have made much of psychiatry obsolete. Psychiatrists are growing tired of watching neurologists, geneticists, immunologists, and microbiologists make dramatic progress in understanding the brain, while the "brain doctors" themselves sit on the sidelines twiddling their thumbs.

These two trends—the increasing disillusionment of psychiatrists with DSM, and the call by psychiatrists for a more scientific approach to the treatment of brain dysfunction—may signal the beginning of the end of the DSM "diagnosis." If so, it won't happen a moment too soon.

CHAPTER 2

The Psychiatric Bible and the Dangers of Misdiagnosis

Some doctors make the same mistakes for twenty years and call it clinical experience.

Dr. Noah Fabricant

Enrichment of the medical vocabulary by the addition of a new name is not always synonymous with enrichment of medical knowledge. New terms for diseases may often serve as camouflage for a lack of understanding.

Petr Skrabanek, Ph.D., and James McCormick, M.D.,
in *Follies and Fallacies in Medicine*

C ONSIDER THE FOLLOWING FOUR PSYCHIATRIC SCENARIOS. Are these examples of (1) the failure of DSM "diagnoses," or (2) state-of-the-art psychiatric care?

1. A 35-year-old woman has terrible nightmares every night for decades, and loses her temper frequently during the day. She sleeps up to 13 hours a night on weekends, and takes frequent long naps. An EEG shows that the woman has abnormal brain wave patterns, and sleep testing reveals that she awakens constantly during the night.

The woman visits a psychiatrist, who gives her the DSM labels of "nightmare disorder" and "primary hypersomnia" (a fancy term for oversleeping). The psychiatrist notes that the cause of her temper outbursts is "hard to explain," and apparently makes no effort to do so. Instead, he prescribes psychotherapy, an antidepressant drug, and a seizure medication. None of these treatments is

27

effective. Lithium reduces the woman's temper outbursts, but only temporarily. After eight months, she becomes discouraged and angry, and leaves treatment.

2. A 46-year-old housewife suffers from severe attacks of dizziness and nausea several nights each week. She reports that during these attacks, the room seems to shimmer and she feels as if she is floating and can't keep her balance. The attacks generally occur in the late afternoon and last for several hours. The patient, after seeing an internist, a neurologist, and an ear-nose-throat specialist (none of whom find anything obvious wrong with her), consults a psychiatrist.

After acknowledging that this patient could have "undiagnosed physical symptoms," the psychiatrist—noting that the patient and her husband have been having marital difficulties, and that the wife's disorder has forced her spouse to take their children out to dinner most evenings—reports that "the context in which these symptoms occur suggests the role of psychological factors in their development." The woman is given a DSM label of "conversion disorder" (hysteria). The psychiatrist's theory is that, by acting crazy, the woman avoids her husband's complaints and gets out of cooking dinner. No effort is made by the psychiatrist to determine whether the woman is experiencing seizures, or suffers from anemia, multiple sclerosis, carbon monoxide poisoning, or any of the many other disorders that can cause dizzy spells.

3. A 20-year-old college student fears he is losing his mind because for two years he has experienced "out-of-body" episodes. During these incidents, his body feels "dead," he often stumbles and loses his balance, and his thoughts seem foggy. At the time of his appointment, the patient is worried because the episodes have increased in frequency to twice a week and are becoming longer in duration.

The student sees a psychiatrist, who gives him the DSM label of "depersonalization disorder"—a label given to people who feel detached or "unreal." The psychiatrist does not report making any physical evaluation to determine whether the patient has seizures or any genetic, metabolic, infectious, drug-related, or neurological disorders that could account for his symptoms.

4. After being exposed to acrid and possibly toxic fumes from a small fire at the dress factory where she works, a 67-year-old woman who has always been outgoing and capable suddenly changes dramatically. She is hospitalized for a week with abdominal pains, nausea, and heart palpitations. These symptoms abate, but after discharge from the hospital she becomes depressed and is frightened to leave her home. She beings having trouble sleeping, and finds herself thinking about her experiences as a concentration camp inmate during World War II.

A psychiatrist refers her for therapy to treat what he labels as posttraumatic stress disorder. After six months of treatment, the woman is still afraid to go to work. No evaluations are performed to determine whether the woman's exposure to fumes from burning synthetic materials and the resulting abdominal pains and heart palpitations are somehow linked to her psychiatric symptoms. In fact, it appears that no physical examination at all is performed by the psychiatrist.

If you're the American Psychiatric Association, you believe these cases represent the best of modern psychiatry. These four examples were taken straight from the *DSM-IV Casebook,* a collection of cases compiled by Robert Spitzer (chairman of a committee that drafted an earlier version of DSM) and colleagues. Presumably, they were selected because the authors believed they were outstanding examples of diagnostic methodology.

But these cases, picked more or less at random from a book designed to teach DSM "diagnosis," clearly reveal the tragedy of DSM. All four of these patients suffer from symptoms indicative of readily diagnosable physical disorders—and all four are in desperate need of true diagnosis. If undiagnosed and untreated, the disorders of several are likely to get worse, not better. One or more of these patients, in my estimation, may be suffering from a potentially fatal illness. Three of them are at serious risk of harming themselves or others while driving or performing other physical tasks that demand unimpaired acuity. At least one of these patients is in danger of losing her job and suffering severe financial hardship because of her symptoms.

Yet little effort has been made to find out what is really wrong with these patients. One has been dismissed as a "hysteric," another has been told she has nightmares and sleep problems (as though she needed to pay hundreds of dollars to find this out!), a third has been given the meaningless label of "depersonalization disorder," and a fourth has been labeled as having a "stress disorder" even though her psychiatrist himself admits that "why such a relatively minor event [a fire] could trigger such an extreme response after so many years is a mystery." But patients don't suffer from "nightmare disorder," or "hypersomnia," or "conversion disorder," or "stress disorder," or "depersonalization disorder." These labels, although they sound impressive, are medically naive. Patients suffer from real brain diseases and dysfunctions, and they need real help. Such help will come not from DSM-oriented doctors playing word games, but only from psychiatrists trained in the science of real differential diagnosis.

Although their numbers have recently begun to increase, psychiatrists practicing such diagnostic detective work are still a rare breed. That's because the DSM cookbook diagnosis method continues to encourage errors in thinking and logic, and has taught psychiatrists a number of sloppy and potentially dangerous habits. Let's examine some of these errors in detail.

DSM Encourages Psychiatrists to Be "Lumpers" Rather than "Splitters"

When I was writing my first book, 30 years ago, I consulted a respected fellow doctor (who was later elected President of the American Psychiatric Association) about the list of diseases I planned to cite as causes of schizophrenia-like symptoms. To my surprise, he was horrified at the suggestion that "schizophrenic" patients actually suffer from a variety of organic disorders. To his way of thinking, our goal as psychiatrists was to fit patients into groups (for instance, "schizophrenics" or "manic depressives"), not to split these groups into individual cases.

This doctor, like many psychiatrists—and especially the authors of DSM—is what I call a "lumper." (In the turn-about-is-fair-play category, I don't have any guilt about labeling the labelers.) The more patients such doctors can stuff into a DSM category, the happier the doctors are. Like doctors in the 1800s, who labeled hundreds of different diseases they didn't understand as "consumption" or "fever," lumpers like to group very dissimilar patients into arbitrary "diagnostic" classifications. "In trying to make logical sense of the classification of mental 'diseases,'" psychiatrist E. Fuller Torrey wrote in *The Death of Psychiatry*, "I have a recurring fantasy of a group of dwarfs sitting in the forest trying to decide whether apples should be classified with tomatoes because they are red, with balls because they are round, with chestnuts because they grow on trees, or with watermelon because they are fruit."

When broad, vague categories won't hold all patients, lumpers simply invent even broader and more vague categories. For instance, when DSM-III's authors found that the label of "autism" was too narrow to include many patients with autism-like symptoms, they created a broader category called "pervasive developmental disorder" (PDD); and when *that* didn't quite cover everyone, DSM-III-R threw in a category called "pervasive developmental disorder not otherwise specified!" This term isn't a diagnosis; it is, as researcher Bernard Rimland notes, "a label concocted by psychiatrists to cover up the fact that they don't know what your child has."

Another wastebasket term in DSM is "mental retardation," a problem that has hundreds of potential causes. Under the "diagnosis" of mental retardation, DSM-IV manages to summarize a number of these causes (Down syndrome, Tay-Sachs disease, tuberous sclerosis, fragile X syndrome, fetal alcohol syndrome, fetal malnutrition, prematurity, lack of oxygen, infections, trauma, lead poisoning, other toxins, and so on) in less than 200 words—without bothering to list the specific symptoms of any of these subcategories. DSM-IV then goes on to discuss the treatment and prognosis of "mental retardation" as though all of these different subcategories require the same interventions and have the same outcomes. But the intervention for a child whose retardation is caused by lead poisoning is very different from the intervention for a child whose retardation is caused by Down syndrome, malnutrition, or an infection. There are reversible, partially reversible, and irreversible forms of mental retardation—something DSM barely mentions.

Lumping is not only inaccurate, but also very dangerous. Let's look at how a particular patient suffers at the hands of lumpers. I'll call our patient, a four-year-old boy, "Johnny."

Johnny's development, up to age four, is normal. A bright, affectionate child, he walks early and talks his parents' ears off. Then—literally overnight—he loses the ability to understand what other people are saying to him. Other changes occur more gradually: Johnny starts avoiding eye contact with other people, stops sleeping at night, and fails to respond to voices and other sounds. He becomes aggressive, sometimes taking swings at his parents. He develops rituals and compulsions, loses his ability to speak, and starts walking with a strange gait.

Johnny's distraught parents are referred to a psychiatrist, who tells them Johnny has many symptoms of autism. But because he doesn't have quite enough symptoms for a cookbook DSM "diagnosis" of autism, the psychiatrist labels him as having pervasive developmental disorder (PDD). He recommends an educational program, and suggests medication to control Johnny's violent behaviors. The parents put Johnny into the program and onto the drugs, but Johnny doesn't improve.

That's because Johnny doesn't have "PDD." He doesn't have "autism," either. He has a rare disorder called Landau-Kleffner syndrome (LKS), which researchers suspect may be caused by infection, immune system dysfunction, or damage to the brain caused by interrupted breathing due to repeated seizures. Medical journals have recently reported that some children with LKS can, if diagnosed early, be successfully treated with corticosteroids or surgery. The disorder can be diagnosed based on a child's medical history, an extensive evaluation, and a specific type of EEG. It can't be diagnosed, or treated, by giving a child a DSM label of autism or PDD—but that's what virtually all children with Landau-Kleffner syndrome receive.

Note that Landau-Kleffner syndrome *itself* isn't a true diagnosis because we don't yet know what causes it. When we pinpoint its exact biological causes, we may be able to develop more effective treatments for the children who have its symptoms. But simply by identifying certain features that occur only in children with LKS (rather than lumping these children in with thousands of other "autistic" children), we've already enhanced our ability to treat or even to cure them. Conversely, if we lumped these children together with thousands of others in a category of symptoms considered "incurable," and waited until their disorder progressed to the stage at which it *was* incurable, we would eliminate any chance they have for a normal life.

Another example of the dangers of lumping, from my own practice, involved a patient named Bobby, a shy eight-year-old with a mop of black hair, the scabby knees of an inveterate baseball player, and well-chewed fingernails. Under his all-American exterior, I discovered a troubled little boy who was failing three of his classes and spending hours each week in detention for "acting out."

"He's not a bad boy," Bobby's mother told me, "but he just flies off the handle. If another child picks on him, Bobby will clobber him—and then immediately feel sorry. He acts first and thinks later." She described Bobby as a jumpy and irritable child who had trouble getting by in school because he tended to "drift off" frequently in class. Another thing that worried her, she said, was that Bobby—who seemed very advanced as a toddler—appeared to be growing more "dull" as he aged.

A previous doctor had labeled Bobby as hyperactive and put him on Ritalin, a popular drug used for children labeled as having hyperactivity and/or attention deficit disorder. Although Bobby took this drug for more than a year, his parents and teachers saw no improvement in his behavior.

Small wonder. When I examined Bobby, and carefully questioned his mother, I learned that he had a number of troubling symptoms, including joint pains and fatigue. I also learned that Bobby ground his teeth at night, walked in his sleep, and regularly wet the bed. I noticed that his neck veins stuck out prominently— a potential sign of heart disease—and that his fingernails (at least what he hadn't chewed off) had ridges suggesting past infection or trauma.

My initial findings led me to conduct an exhaustive evaluation that turned up not one, but several causes of Bobby's symptoms. He had an abnormal EEG, indicating that he suffered from frequent mild seizures. Laboratory tests revealed that his lead levels were significantly elevated, and that his joint pains were due to a previous "strep" infection. In addition, his red blood cell count was abnormal and there was a suggestion of a cardiac problem.

Bobby's diagnosis isn't complete yet, because I'm still narrowing down which of his many problems is causing each of his symptoms. I'm treating his seizures, his elevated lead levels, and his joint pain. I've also referred him to a cardiologist to see how serious his heart problem is. I'm monitoring his abnormal blood cell count to see whether it is a chronic symptom indicating yet more biological problems, or only reflective of his lead poisoning. In short, I'm doing my best to uncover all of the many causes of Bobby's troubles, rather than just giving all of them one convenient label. Splitting, unlike lumping, is an ongoing and ever-evolving process.

Bobby, like Johnny, was suffering from treatable problems. In both cases, the problems were serious and would most likely have gotten worse over time if not diagnosed and treated. "Lumpers" would have shoehorned both children into categories based on DSM symptoms, rather than diagnosing them as individuals. For patients with serious diseases, this can be a fatal mistake.

Lumping can be a dangerous mistake even for patients with no disease at all. Lilian, a 46-year-old woman, came to me with a troubling problem: she'd gradually grown sad and weary, and just getting through the day was now difficult. A jogger and self-described health nut, Lilian told me, "I just don't understand why this is happening to me of all people." She told me she felt drained by the middle of the day, had terrible trouble concentrating on her work—a major problem for an accountant—and was so tired at night that "I can barely get up the stairs to bed." I believed her: the way she sagged in her chair, the dark circles under her eyes, and the lack of sparkle in her eyes all told me that Lilian was running on empty and desperately needed help.

Unfortunately, she hadn't gotten any help from her previous psychiatrist. He hadn't asked why this formerly vivacious, athletic woman had gradually become so "down in the dumps"; instead, he simply prescribed Paxil, an antidepressant medication. After all, Lilian had enough symptoms to be lumped into the DSM category of "depression"—and that was all he needed to know.

But Lilian didn't need medication; she needed a good night's sleep. It turned out that her husband's chronic and horrific snoring had been waking her every five to ten minutes during the night, disrupting her sleep patterns and leaving her groggy and despondent. After six years of constantly interrupted sleep, Lilian was suffering from a severe case of sleep deprivation—a condition that can cause intense despondency, fatigue, and even disorientation and hallucinations. My prescription: "Stop taking antidepressants, send your husband to a sleep clinic for treatment, and make him sleep in the guest room for now." By asking questions about Lilian's personal situation—rather than lumping her in with all other "depressed" patients—I was able to avoid treating *her* for her husband's medical problem!

One of the chief dangers of lumping is that it encourages "one-size-fits-all" treatment. Almost all "depressed" patients get anti-depressants and psychotherapy, even though some really have lupus, other have low thyroid hormone levels, and still others have Lyme disease—and some, like Lilian, have nothing wrong with them at all. Almost all "schizophrenics" get psychotropic drugs, even though some are suffering from brain tumors, or heavy-metal toxicity, or reactions to prescription medications. Almost all "hyperactive" children get Ritalin, even though they may actually suffer from lead poisoning, worms, or cardiac problems. In other words, patients are tailored to fit available treatments—instead of treatments being tailored for individual patients.

This misguided approach reminds me of the fable about the king who decided that his shoemakers could make more shoes if all of the shoes were the same size and style. It sounded like a great idea. The only problem was that 92 out of every 100 people in the king's country had to go barefoot for the rest of their lives, because the "average" size shoe didn't fit them.

Unlike lumpers, splitters look at each patient as an individual—not as a member of a DSM category. This approach helps ensure that patients receive accurate diagnoses and appropriate treatment. A psychiatrist who views 100 "depressed" patients as 100 individuals who potentially have 100 different diagnoses will cure far more of them than a psychiatrist who gives all 100 patients the same DSM label and treats them with Prozac. Likewise, a doctor who discovers the reasons for patients' anxiety attacks will cure more of these patients than the very successful psychiatrist in my town who recently said, "Anxiety *is* a diagnosis"—suggesting that one need look no further than the DSM label.

Besides being the exact opposite of correct diagnostic technique, lumping has another serious drawback: it muddies and distorts research findings. Doctors studying the causes of schizophrenia, for example, won't learn much if their 30 study subjects actually suffer from 30 different disorders. The use of vague DSM categories to select study subjects—the approach used in most psychiatric research today—virtually guarantees that research findings will be misleading and will point future researchers in wrong directions.

DSM Teaches Psychiatrists to Look at the Book—Not at the Patient

Making a diagnosis is a lot like solving a crime. The doctor begins with an almost endless list of "suspects"—diseases, injuries, toxins, infections. By asking the right questions, the doctor narrows down the list of suspects. The next step is to collect evidence and then reevaluate the list of suspects, crossing off those for whom the tests provide alibis. Eventually, in most cases, the doctor will discover the right culprit (or culprits). And, just as in a Sherlock Holmes mystery, that culprit often is a surprise—if the doctor doesn't make up his or her mind before all the facts are in.

But DSM teaches a psychiatrist to pick a label first—as soon as he or she can identify enough symptoms to wedge a patient into a DSM category—and ask questions later (or not at all). Proper diagnosis is based largely on observation and curiosity ("Why would this incoherent patient also have a low-grade fever and a rash?"). DSM, on the other hand, actually trains doctors to *ignore* major medical clues, by offering canned symptom lists and encouraging doctors to push patients into them. In effect, it says, "Ignore any symptom that doesn't fit the picture." Thus, the incoherent patient is labeled as having "dementia" or "schizophrenia"—never mind that she also has a rash and low-grade fever. The aggressive patient is labeled as having "antisocial personality disorder"—even when there are marks on his legs from steroid needles. The weeping patient is labeled as "depressed," and her enlarged thyroid gland is not examined. To make nondiagnosis even easier, most DSM categories end with a "not otherwise specified" category—

a grab-bag label for patients who don't fit any other category. Thus, a patient with puzzling symptoms can actually wind up "diagnosed" as "personality disorder not otherwise specified," "delirium not otherwise specified," or "psychotic disorder not otherwise specified." This system is about as useful as labeling a cancer patient with unusual symptoms as having a "lump disorder not otherwise specified."

A tragic example of such diagnostic tunnel vision, cited by therapist Paula Caplan in *They Say You're Crazy,* involved a young boy admitted to a Canadian hospital after he began vomiting repeatedly. After what must have been a very brief and limited evaluation, the boy was turned over to a psychiatrist. "The outcome of that consultation," Caplan says, "was an assertion that the vomiting was psychologically caused and a recommendation that the staff make the child clean up his own vomit as a way of teaching him to stop." But this treatment program, no doubt based on a pat DSM or ICD label of "mental" disorder, proved to be fatal. The child, who suffered from a bowel blockage, died shortly after being "diagnosed" by the psychiatrist.

This case is particularly horrifying because the child's condition was common, easily diagnosable, and completely treatable. Intestinal blockage, which causes bloating, constipation or diarrhea, and, eventually, excruciating pain and shock, can be readily diagnosed with a barium swallow, and doctors can make a preliminary diagnosis simply by palpating the abdomen and listening for abnormal bowel sounds. Yet the doctors in this case, and apparently the hospital staff as well, overlooked the dramatic symptoms this child must have been suffering, and focused instead on a "mental" problem he never had—simply because a psychiatrist identified the child's problem as being "all in his head."

Psychiatric training should teach physicians not to ignore atypical symptoms, but to search for them. Abnormal hair growth, weight problems, skin discolorations, bad fingernails, unusual eye color, abnormal gait, strange posture, or peculiar facial expressions can steer a medical detective toward a diagnosis. These clues, not a cookbook list of symptoms, are what solve medical mysteries.

There are thousands of such clues. Suppose, for instance, that you have odd ridges on your fingernails. Those are called "Beau's lines," and they tell me to check you for cardiac problems, past infections, or physical trauma. (Fingernails, incidentally, are much like the rings of a tree trunk: they tell a great deal about a patient's history.) Or suppose you've developed a "buffalo hump" on your back, a ruddy complexion, and a pot belly. You may have Cushing's syndrome, a disorder caused by excessive production of a hormone called cortisone. Protruding eyes? I'll check you for an overactive thyroid. Dry skin and thin hair? I'll check for the opposite condition—hypothyroidism. The list is almost endless, but the moral is simple: every unusual symptom is a signpost pointing toward a diagnosis. A doctor who follows these signs will generally arrive at the correct destination; one who ignores them will be, diagnostically speaking, lost in the woods.

A good example of the importance of physical clues in making a diagnosis is Wilson's disease (hepatolenticular degeneration). This genetic disorder causes copper to accumulate in the body tissues—particularly the liver and brain—and can lead to severe liver disease, tremor, rigid muscles, and dementia. Behavioral symptoms, which can range from sexual exhibitionism to psychosis, often occur well before signs of liver disease are apparent. (In one study I conducted, 100 percent of 25 patients with Wilson's disease showed behavioral abnormalities before organ damage was detectable.) Psychiatrists often give such patients pat DSM labels, without bothering to do careful exams; in doing so, they condemn many to death from hepatitis or cirrhosis. "In 37 of our patients who presented primarily with neurologic symptoms," physicians George Brewer and Vilma Yuzbasiyan-Gurkan recently reported in *Medicine,* "approximately two-thirds had psychiatric difficulties before the diagnosis was made." In all, almost half of these patients had enough behavioral symptoms to require psychiatric treatment. But their disease went undiagnosed, even though Wilson's disease is a well-known disorder that all psychiatrists learn about in medical school.

Because of the subtle but detectable physical signs of Wilson's disease, there is little excuse for such misdiagnosis. These signs include an odd smiling appearance, acne, thinning skin, and—the most remarkable sign—Kayser-Fleischer rings, which are green or golden-brown rings around the cornea of the eye. In many cases, an alert psychiatrist can make a tentative diagnosis of Wilson's disease within minutes of meeting a patient. (A careful evaluation is then needed, of course, to confirm the diagnosis.)

A few months ago, I treated a very troubled 40-year-old man named Bob. Running his hands through his stringy blond hair, Bob told me he was convinced that everyone was out to get him: his boss, the residents at the apartment complex where he worked, the police, even total strangers. He complained that people called him a "weirdo," because he got shaky and heard voices when women tried to talk to him. "They talk about me a lot," he said. "They tell the lifeguards at the beach where I swim that there's a pervert in the parking lot." Bob had held a series of low-paying jobs, but they usually didn't last long because he angered or frightened his coworkers. At the time I interviewed him, he was sleeping in his truck.

Bob had previously been seen for two hours by another psychiatrist, who gave him a whole slew of DSM labels including "psychotic disorder not otherwise specified," possible "schizophrenia," and possible "bipolar mood disorder in mixed state." The doctor's report contained no evidence of any medical evaluation (other than a handful of questions he had asked Bob about past diseases), laboratory evaluations, brain scans, or other diagnostic inquiries. In the section of his "diagnosis" where the psychiatrist was to include any physical disorders, he had listed "none."

This psychiatrist had lots of vague theories about the causes of Bob's problems: a dysfunctional family, Bob's early loss of his biological mother (who died of cancer when he was a child), a disapproving stepmother. What the doctor didn't have, however, was a clue about what really ailed Bob. I know, because I diagnosed Bob shortly afterward as having Wilson's disease. Bob's paranoid behavior, his unusual sexual interests, and his increasingly erratic behavior were common symptoms seen in patients with Wilson's disease. But the most obvious tip-off was the odd pigmentation of Bob's eyes—something his previous psychiatrist had missed altogether.

I've diagnosed many patients by pursuing similar clues. One was Danny, a bright sandy-haired nine-year-old with a "Huck Finn" personality and a mischievous twinkle in his eyes, who'd been labeled as hyperactive because of his fidgeting and disruptive classroom behavior. Danny was a playground leader and a first-rate class clown who excelled at starting spit-wad battles and cafeteria food fights, but when it came to academic work—or to sitting still—he was a total failure. He'd been placed in a special education class after his teachers noticed that he reversed letters like "b" and "d," and sometimes began reading or writing from the wrong side of the page. His parents, who assumed that he suffered from attention deficit disorder and, possibly, dyslexia, were seeking a prescription for Ritalin, hoping that it would improve his behavior and his school performance.

A major clue to Danny's problem was his hair: the whorl (the little "swirly" patch of hair at the crown of the head), was in the middle, rather than in the normal location on the side of the head opposite from the dominant hand. I also discovered that Danny used his right hand for writing, but kicked a football with his left foot and used his left hand for eating. In addition, his left eye was dominant, and he had difficulty distinguishing right from left.

After ruling out other possible disorders, I diagnosed Danny as having mixed dominance, in which neither side of the brain is clearly dominant. This can cause reading and writing difficulties and poor school performance, which in turn can lead to irritability and frustration—or, as in Danny's case, can cause a child to compensate by becoming an athlete or a class clown. I referred Danny to a reading clinic, which taught him techniques for dealing with his mixed dominance. Within eight weeks he was able to return to a regular classroom, and he later became one of the top students in his class.

Medical clues like Bob's eye rings and Danny's hair whorl are often overlooked by DSM-oriented psychiatrists. This is a serious failing: a physician trained to ignore such obvious symptoms, or to write them off as "atypical" rather than investigating their causes, is diagnostically crippled, and frequently endangers his or her patients.

So, for that matter, does a physician who asks patients only enough questions to generate sufficient symptoms for a DSM label. Patients are gold mines of information to a doctor who's willing to listen. One of the most valuable tools I use in my diagnostic endeavors is a "24-hour-day" profile, which traces a patient's activities and symptoms throughout the day. This technique gives me many clues about a patient's life and the possible nature of his or her illness. By carefully taking a patient through an entire day's worth of activities, both waking and sleeping, I learn vital diagnostic information that won't show up on a DSM symptom list. For instance:

- *Does the patient have daily routines or habits?* I recently talked with a father whose young "hyperactive" son regularly stands on his head, saying it makes him feel better. This habit raises questions about inner-ear problems—or perhaps cardiac disease. Other habits, such as constant throat-clearing or the habit of sleeping with four or more pillows, also may point to physical disorders.

- *How does the patient sleep?* Frequent waking to urinate during the night may indicate incipient diabetes. Fatigue, sadness, despair, hostility, and anxiety may stem from sleep apnea, a serious disorder in which patients actually stop breathing numerous times during the night. (Potentially fatal, sleep apnea can now be cured by surgery.) And sleepwalking is a definite sign that something significant, and quite likely life-threatening, is wrong with the brain.

- *Does the patient dream?* I'm not interested in the content of dreams—that's the Freudians' department. But I am interested in whether a patient dreams at all. And, if a patient speaks more than one language, I'm curious about which language is spoken in the dreams. A patient who has become fluent in a second language, and now speaks that language all day, should dream in that language as well. A patient from Greece who has spoken and dreamed in English for decades, but suddenly begins dreaming in Greek again, may be showing signs of a brain dysfunction.

- *Does the patient have hobbies?* A gun enthusiast who frequents shooting ranges and makes his or her own bullets is at risk of developing behavioral problems due to either lead poisoning or nitrate toxicity, which can cause severe headaches, insomnia, and other problems commonly dismissed as "hypochondriasis." Artists are exposed to cadmium, solvents, and other toxins that can provoke brain dysfunction. A recent report suggests that some divers suffer brain lesions caused by small gas bubbles released into the bloodstream during dives. And people who frequently skateboard, roller-skate, play contact sports, or go bungee-jumping are prone to head injuries that can impair thinking and behavior. (I suspect head trauma in any patients involved regularly in such activities, even if they don't report major head injuries, because even seemingly mild head bumps can cause concussions.)

- *Where does the patient work?* Do any coworkers experience symptoms similar to the patient's? Does the patient's job involve chemicals or toxins? Does it expose the patient to viral or bacterial infections (i.e., a hospital job)? A surprising range of brain dysfunctions, many of them serious, stem from exposure to toxic or infectious agents at work. Veterinarians, for instance, run a higher-than-normal risk of contracting brucellosis, a bacterial infection that is transmissible from animals to humans and can cause persistent sadness, impotence, insomnia, and psychosis.

- *What vitamins or minerals does the patient take?* Vitamin/ mineral supplements are generally harmless and often therapeutic, but excessive intakes of some nutrients can cause neurological symptoms. I once diagnosed a young girl whose seizures, behavior problems, bone pain, and dry and kinky hair were caused by excessive intake of vitamin A. Overdoses of vitamin D can also cause "mental" symptoms such as fatigue, despondency, and even psychosis. Conversely, a poor diet low in vitamins or minerals can cause severe behavioral disorders; iron deficiency, for instance, can cause irritability, fatigue, and symptoms labeled as "conduct disorder" or "hyperactivity."

- *Does the patient eat unusual foods, eat too much or too little, or have unusual reactions to any foods?* Eating habits can indicate allergies, anemia, and other conditions that can cause severe "mental" symptoms. For instance, my 24-hour-day profile of a 31-year-old female patient, labeled as a "hysteric" by previous doctors, uncovered eating habits and fatigue patterns that suggested neuroglycopenia (chronic low blood sugar severe enough to impair brain function, causing intellectual deterioration and marked personality changes). Tests confirmed my suspicions, and the problem was readily corrected. Even temporary dietary changes can point to a diagnosis. Physician Siegfried Kra, in *Aging Myths,* reported the case of an 80-year-old woman who suddenly developed memory loss and despondency. It turned out her heart problem, a condition that had been controlled fairly well, had worsened after she consumed a salty Polish ham given to her as a Christmas present!

In addition to doing a 24-hour-day profile, I ask patients to tell me about any notable experiences—both recent and past—in their lives. Often, in these experiences, I uncover clues that unravel the entire mystery of a patient's disease. For instance, a patient who frequently hikes in the woods, particularly in the Northeast, may have Lyme disease, a tick-borne disease that can cause memory loss, mood swings, sleep problems, and even dementia. Someone new to the Southwest may have Valley fever, a fungal disease endemic to the area, which can lead to severe fatigue and despondency. A traveler just back from Africa or South America may have cysticercosis, which can cause delusions, dementia, assaultive behavior, suicidal behavior, and symptoms resembling schizophrenia. And a person who has recently handled pigeons or other birds may have cryptococcosis or psittacosis, bird-borne diseases that can cause psychosis. Most of the details learned in the course of questioning are irrelevant, but the doctor who sifts through them carefully almost always finds a few diagnostic gems.

To quote an old (but true) cliché, patients don't walk into a doctor's office with their diagnoses written on their foreheads. However, many patients do have their diagnoses "written" all over them—if a physician is smart enough to know where to look. Many patients will tell the physician what's wrong with them, if he or she listens carefully for the clues they provide. Unfortunately, psychiatrists trained in DSM "diagnosis" often aren't looking *or* listening carefully enough.

DSM Encourages Psychiatrists to Be Lazy

Just as doctors don't need to look carefully at patients to make DSM diagnoses, they also don't need to bother with extensive exams, tests, follow-up evaluations, and all of the work that goes into pinpointing the exact cause of a disorder. They can simply pick symptoms that fit a DSM label, write a prescription, recommend a psychotherapist, and be done with their patients.

To show how this works, let's borrow again from the "state-of-the-art" *DSM-IV Casebook*. The very first case in this teaching manual concerns a patient called Celia, who has been brought to an emergency room in handcuffs and leg chains after "going wild" and trying to bite people. She doesn't remember doing any of this, but says such attacks have happened before. Her relatives say that during the attacks she screams, kicks, bites, and sometimes tries to cut herself with a knife.

The attending psychiatrist who talks to her in the emergency room learns that the woman was raped repeatedly by her uncle in her childhood. She currently has difficulty sleeping, and often has bad dreams. She is usually sad, and has vague suicidal thoughts. She spends most of her time watching TV, and has failed to finish school or keep a job. In addition, she has a history of drug abuse.

A number of Celia's symptoms, the doctor admits, could suggest temporal lobe seizures. (Such seizures are sometimes associated with bizarre and violent behavior that the patient does not remember afterward.) This condition would be highly consistent with her sleep problems, her inability to finish school or hold a job, and her irritability. But is the woman checked by the psychiatrist for seizures? Is she given a 24-hour EEG? Is she tested for other problems that can resemble seizures, such as disoriented states accompanying low blood sugar? Is her history of drug abuse explored thoroughly?

Apparently not, because no mention is made of any physical examination or tests. But then, there's no *need* for an examination or tests, because the woman's symptoms also conveniently fit a DSM-IV "diagnosis" of posttraumatic stress disorder (PTSD)—a label frequently applied to patients who have suffered any sort of significant emotional trauma in the past. (The public is most familiar with this label as a description of Vietnam War veterans, but it's rapidly becoming one of the most common DSM "diagnoses" for patients in general, because it's easy to apply. After all, every patient who sees a psychiatrist has, at one time or another, suffered an emotional trauma!)

Under DSM, the fact that Celia was raped in childhood "trumps" any other diagnostic clues and renders them inconsequential. Thus, she is quickly labeled as having PTSD, sent home from the hospital, and scheduled for psychotherapy. "For reasons that are not clear," the authors of the *DSM-IV Casebook* say, "the follow-up plan did not work," and the patient—who was back in the emergency room two weeks later—did not keep her therapy appointments. No attempt appears to have been made to follow up on her case, but it's a good bet that Celia's bizarre behaviors have continued to occur.

This is not medicine. Medicine consists of finding the right diagnosis, not just the most convenient label. Until this patient received a thorough examination, a 24-hour EEG, a blood sugar test, and numerous other evaluations, her psychiatrists couldn't begin to guess what was wrong with her. In my opinion, telling this woman that her symptoms were "all in her head" and prescribing psychotherapy, in the absence of a real diagnosis, was equivalent to nontreatment—a very dangerous situation, in light of the patient's life-threatening behavior.

Unfortunately, such pat labels are all too common. Most of the patients who come to me after seeing other doctors have received little or no evaluation beyond a few tests designed to forestall malpractice suits. Many patients with seizure-causing disorders, for instance, have received DSM labels without ever having had a single EEG. Many diabetic patients have never had a glucose test, and many iron-deficient patients have never had a test for anemia. And I've diagnosed patients with brain tumors who had never been given a brain scan—and even a couple of patients whose brain scans *did* show tumors that were overlooked. All of these patients, of course, had received earlier "diagnoses"—straight from DSM.

In some instances, I can feel for the psychiatrists involved. When one gets used to thinking of every patient as having a DSM "mental" disorder, it's all too easy to develop a mind-set that excludes any other causes—even when they're staring you in the face. In his book *The New Psychiatry,* Jerrold Maxmen offers a typical example, calling it "one of my least proud moments during my training." While in the emergency room, he was asked to evaluate an unhappy patient with a blank expression and a slow gait. Recognizing DSM symptoms of "major depression," Maxmen had the patient admitted with this DSM label. A hospital staff member called him some time later to explain that the man's symptoms were due not to "depression" but to Parkinson's disease, a disorder that causes motor and behavioral disturbances. "I erred," Maxmen says, "by not questioning my first impression and by not systematically considering every other diagnostic possibility."

Such misdiagnoses will continue to be common until psychiatry replaces its emphasis on quick DSM labeling with an emphasis on intellectual curiosity and hard investigative work. Because of the powerful hold DSM has on insurance companies, psychiatric hospitals, and training programs for future psychiatrists, change won't come easily. (I should know; I've been after the profession for 30 years.) In the meantime, the onus is on the patient, to seek second opinions and to question DSM labels.

DSM Fosters Stagnation

Doctors trained to use DSM don't have to keep up with the medical literature. Depression is depression is depression, until the next revision of DSM calls it something else.

Making accurate diagnoses however, requires keeping up with medical developments. New genetic tests, for instance, make it possible to pinpoint many disorders—but a doctor who isn't familiar with these tests won't know when to consult with a geneticist. New brain imaging technologies are being developed every year, but a doctor who doesn't understand MRI, PET, or SPECT tests may not know which ones to order. A physician doesn't need to know the nitty-gritty of these tests, but he or she *does* need to know the usefulness, limitations, and confidence levels of each.

Furthermore, the world outside of medicine changes—and each change alters patterns of diseases and brain dysfunctions. Twenty years ago, for instance, travel to and from faraway countries was rare. But immigration and travel patterns have changed, and modern American psychiatrists may encounter medical problems once seen only in remote African villages or rural Chinese communities. Sleeping sickness, malaria, filariasis, and rat lung worm all have gone from being interesting case studies in psychiatric textbooks to being distinct diagnostic possibilities—although you won't learn much about any of them from DSM. Patterns of domestic disease change, as well; in fact, there's intriguing new evidence that the prevalence of symptoms labeled as "schizophrenia" may be related to the spread of the species of ticks that carry Lyme disease and tick-borne encephalitis, and that the Borna disease virus—which affects horses and cows—may also cause depression and personality disorders in humans.

Psychiatrists who rely strictly on DSM frequently don't keep up with such developments. (After all, if you simply label all patients with feelings of sadness and hopelessness as "depressed," why worry about what *causes* the depression?) In addition, these psychiatrists often don't *un*learn old ideas that science has debunked. For instance, PET scans and other new technologies are revealing marked abnormalities in the brains of psychopaths, once thought to be victims of bad upbringing. The behavioral symptoms DSM labels as "borderline personality disorder"—lack of empathy, suicidal or self-injurious behavior, feelings of emptiness, and poor relational skills—have recently been linked to abnormal levels of the brain chemical serotonin. And sexual disorders such as pedophilia and exhibitionism, almost universally considered by psychiatrists to be caused by upbringing, are now known to have a number of physical causes, including tumors and Wilson's disease. Psychiatrists who believe in correctly diagnosing their patients' medical conditions make a point of keeping up with recent medical developments by reading not only the psychiatric literature, but also research from neurology, molecular biology, and other medical fields. But psychiatrists who rely on DSM labeling, rather than keeping up with changes in medicine, will fall farther behind each year and do more and more damage.

This is true not only of individual psychiatrists but of our entire field. While other medical specialties have been enjoying revolutionary advances because of research into genetics, immunology, molecular biology, and new diagnostic technologies, psychiatry has spent decades refining and rewriting its system of labeling. Huge amounts of time and money have been wasted on research into the reliability of DSM. Such research doesn't advance medical science; it simply determines whether 100 psychiatrists, given the same list of symptoms, will apply the same DSM label to 100 different patients. Funds desperately needed to investigate the roots of brain dysfunction have instead been spent on what is essentially a word game (Will Dr. X call it "borderline personality"? Will Dr. Y call it "dissociative disorder"?). This obsession with labeling contributes nothing to our understanding of disease processes.

The hours other medical specialists are able to spend learning new diagnostic and treatment procedures are frequently spent by psychiatrists simply trying to figure out how to apply DSM labels. "No argument I might make about the bankruptcy of DSM-III and its offspring could be as powerful as [psychiatrists'] own experience with case conferences," psychiatrist Matthew P. Dumont wrote in the journal *Readings*. "Who can calculate the wasted hours of foolish, futile discussion about how to compartmentalize patients who never seem to fit the numbered cubicles in which we are forced . . . to place them?" Physicians have few enough hours to read journals or attend seminars, without wasting many of them learning the difference between "adjustment disorder unspecified" and "adjustment disorder with mixed disturbance of emotions and conduct."

Given that much of a psychiatrist's training and continuing education consists of learning to use the DSM, and that a large percentage of research in the field is given over to analyzing DSM labels, it's little wonder that of all the medical sciences, psychiatry has reported the fewest breakthroughs in diagnosis and treatment. Most developments in the treatment of brain dysfunction, in fact, have come from other fields such as neurology, genetics, and immunology. Luckily for them, they have no DSM.

*   *   *

DSM teaches psychiatrists to lump and label rather than to split and diagnose. It teaches them to disregard important symptoms that don't fit conveniently into a DSM list, to ignore patients, and to skip the scutwork of diagnosis—often with disastrous consequences. DSM leaves psychiatrists on the outskirts of the dramatic progress currently being made in molecular biology, immunology, and other fields of medicine.

But there are even greater dangers from DSM; we'll look at them in the next few chapters. The most troubling is that DSM has led to the unnecessary drugging of millions of Americans who could be diagnosed, treated, and cured without the use of toxic and potentially lethal medications.

CHAPTER 3

Bad Medicine

Treating the Symptoms and Ignoring the Causes

There are some remedies worse than the disease.

Publius Syrus, first century B.C.

If I give you a pill, I am really not treating your problem. You will go away, but your problems will not.

Dr. Joseph A. Pursch, U.S.N.

I WAS VISITED RECENTLY BY JOHN, AN UP-AND-COMING YOUNG engineer with two children and a high-paying job at a growing computer firm. John's future had looked rosy, with a promotion and a big raise in the offing. He and his wife, Annie, were talking about buying a big house in the suburbs, getting a dog, and taking a second honeymoon in Europe. John and Annie went camping with the kids, played softball on his company team, and took ballroom dancing lessons together. Their friends referred to them, jokingly, as "Ozzie and Harriet."

Then, gradually, John began suffering from unexplainable sadness and overwhelming fatigue. He cut down on his overtime hours, and slept in on the weekends, but his weariness became more and more debilitating. He was finding it impossible to concentrate on his work at the office, and was losing control of his emotions; just the week before, during a candlelight dinner with Annie at a fancy restaurant, he'd broken down and spent an hour sobbing uncontrollably in the restroom. "I'm going to pieces," he said simply. "My wife can't take much more—and neither can I."

Neither could John's boss, who was becoming angry at his poor productivity and his fits of weeping, and was threatening to demote him to another job—or fire him altogether. Over the past two years, John had gone from being happy and successful to being a despondent wreck in danger of losing his job and his family.

Annie, a plump, attractive brunette who came with John to his first appointment, told me that the onset of his symptoms had been insidious. "He was very close to one of his uncles," she told me, "and a few months after Uncle Jack died, John started seeming moody. I just assumed it was grief, and that he'd get over it with time. But the more time passed, the worse John got." Now, she said, she wouldn't even leave him home alone, for fear that he might try to kill himself. She'd flushed most of his medications down the toilet, because she worried—with good reason—that the psychotropic drugs that weren't curing him could be more effective in taking his life.

It was Annie, in fact, who insisted that John make an appointment to see me. I was John's fourth choice as a doctor—he'd already visited a general practitioner and two psychiatrists—but, luckily for John, his wife was a persistent woman. John's previous doctors had saddled him with a variety of DSM labels and treated him with 26 different medications, without ever conducting a single neurological examination. If they had, they would have discovered—as I did, after conducting a thorough diagnostic evaluation—that he suffered from a slow-growing meningioma (a tumor of the brain lining). When I broke the news to John and Annie, she said, simply, "I never thought that a brain tumor could be good news."

John's tumor was removed, and his sadness and fatigue rapidly cleared. Because the tumor was benign, John's prognosis is excellent. He and Annie have bought their dream house, and they're back in dance class again. John is a lucky man; if he'd continued with the various drug treatments prescribed by his other physicians, his tumor would have continued to grow and eventually would have become inoperable.

What Drugs Can—and Can't—Do

John's story illustrates one of the most dangerous false beliefs of modern psychiatry—the belief that *masking symptoms with drugs is equivalent to treating disease.* More than twenty million Americans take Prozac, Ritalin, Xanax, Valium, or other potent psychotropic (brain-altering) drugs prescribed on the basis of DSM labels. Most of these patients—and their physicians—honestly believe that these drugs constitute "treatment." But many of these patients would be better off receiving *no treatment at all* than taking drugs.

Let me stress, before going on, that some drugs are invaluable in treating brain dysfunction. Antibiotics can kill infectious agents that affect the brain, such as syphilis and rickettsia. Replacement drugs, such as insulin or thyroid hormone or dopamine, can successfully treat chemical imbalances. And cardiac drugs, prescribed for heart problems that cause anxiety and other behavioral symptoms, can literally be lifesavers.

Other drugs can control the symptoms of patients with disorders we can't yet successfully treat. Occasionally, for instance, I put patients on anticonvulsants while I rule out possible treatable disorders that can cause seizures. Or I prescribe pain-killing medication for patients with inoperable tumors, when symptomatic relief is all that is possible.

Even neuroleptic (literally, "nerve-seizing") drugs, although they're terribly dangerous, are called for in some cases. Many individuals labeled as retarded or psychotic can't yet be effectively treated, even when we understand the roots of their disorders. Children with Lesch-Nyhan syndrome are a good example: we know that their behavior problems, which can include chewing off their own fingers, are caused by a genetic defect, but we can't yet *treat* that defect. And although we're pinpointing more and more genetic, metabolic, and immune system abnormalities in individuals labeled as "autistic" or "schizophrenic," we can't yet cure the majority of them. Some of these individuals exhibit behavior so bizarre and violent that it endangers them or the people around them; in such cases, neuroleptic drug use may be justified, and indeed necessary, for the sake of the patients and their families. For those "schizophrenics" whose brain dysfunctions can't yet be identified, neuroleptic drugs can often make it possible to lead near-normal lives—although always with the risk of severe drug side effects. At the moment, this is as close as medical science can get to a cure.

Still another valid use for drugs is in a diagnostic technique called a "therapeutic challenge." By giving a patient a brief trial of a drug and noting its effects, a doctor can often gain valuable clues about the origins of behavioral symptoms. In these cases, the drug is *not a treatment but a diagnostic tool.* If a patient responds to a brief trial of an antidepressant, for instance, that doesn't tell the physician that he or she should prescribe the drug; rather, it tells the physician to investigate the areas of the brain that the antidepressant affects.

As a physician with advanced training in pharmacology, I'm not opposed to the careful use of drugs to diagnose, treat, or cure behavioral problems. What I *do* oppose is the use of powerful and dangerous drugs such as Prozac, Haldol, and Ritalin as chemical straitjackets *in cases where diagnosis is possible and effective treatments, or even cures, exist.*

Psychotropic drugs don't cure brain dysfunction. Their sole purpose is to suppress symptoms. But *a symptom is a signal that something is wrong,* and ignoring or suppressing it won't make the problem go away. If your smoke alarm goes off in the middle of the night, do you check to see whether there's a fire—or do you simply disconnect the smoke alarm and go back to bed? Physicians using powerful drugs to mask symptoms of disease are, in effect, disconnecting the body's alarm systems and allowing disease processes to continue disrupting the brain. Because the brain is one of the body's most sensitive organs, it's often the first to send a warning signal that something is seriously wrong with the body. Ignoring such signals can be dangerous or even fatal.

To fully understand how ludicrous the DSM-and-drug approach is, imagine what would happen if physicians in other fields simply gave patients symptom-masking drugs instead of diagnosing and treating them. Picture, for instance, a patient visiting a general practitioner for treatment of a swollen hand. A quick evaluation by the physician reveals that the hand indeed is twice its normal size, feels hot, and is turning an unpleasant color. Now suppose that the physician—instead of diagnosing the patient's life-threatening infection and treating the infection with antibiotics—simply prescribes pain-killing drugs and sends the patient home! "Treating" a patient's behavioral symptoms with Prozac and Ritalin is no different. Although the patient may be lulled into a temporary sense of wellness, the disease processes that created the patient's symptoms are still present and often are growing worse.

Consider the case of Mona, a woman I once treated, who was labeled as "psychotic" in early adulthood. A model-thin beauty with high cheekbones and distinctive almond eyes, Mona had married a successful attorney shortly after leaving college. But her husband soon began spending long hours at the office to avoid his new bride's "crazy" behavior, which included screaming at him, physically attacking him, and even hallucinating. By the time she'd been married a year, Mona had gained several dress sizes—even though she hardly ever ate. She'd become slovenly, no longer took care of the house, and often drank until she passed out on the sofa.

For the next 25 years, a local psychiatrist treated Mona with one drug after another—the accepted treatment for her DSM labels of "major depression" and "atypical psychosis"—but she grew progressively worse. Her marriage dissolved, and her drinking (which had been a problem even before the onset of psychotic behavior) grew increasingly worse. Finally, a neighbor suggested that Mona make an appointment with me. When my comprehensive evaluation showed that she had elevated calcium levels, she said, "I've been told that for years."

Her doctors may have told her—but they didn't do anything about it. It was an astounding oversight on their part, because elevated calcium can be a sign of high parathyroid hormone levels, which in turn can indicate tumors or parathyroid disease—either of which could have explained Mona's bizarre behaviors. Parathyroid disorders can cause a wide range of symptoms, including weight gain, despondency, anxiety, memory loss, hallucinations, and dementia.

As I suspected, further evaluation revealed that Mona had a parathyroid tumor; when it was removed, her symptoms improved markedly. (Although she's now in much better shape than before the surgery, Mona still suffers from some "mental" problems— probably a result of her alcoholism. One might wonder whether her drinking problem was exacerbated by her despair during 25 years of failed drug treatment. One also might wonder what this intelligent, attractive woman could have done with her life if she'd been diagnosed when her tumor first developed.)

Mona is only one of millions of patients whose medications are covering up undiagnosed disease. Among them are thousands of people (most of them women) who suffer from systemic lupus erythematosus, or SLE. Lupus is an autoimmune disorder—that is, a disease in which the immune system goes haywire and the body mistakenly attacks its own cells. SLE, a very serious form of lupus, is potentially fatal; but although it can't yet be cured, it can be managed with appropriate therapy. The life expectancy of SLE patients has increased greatly over the past few decades because cases are being diagnosed earlier, allowing for prompt treatment—particularly treatment of the kidney problems SLE often causes.

But SLE patients don't always get diagnosed early, because many people with SLE develop psychiatric symptoms before other symptoms (including fever, malaise, joint pain, and a characteristic butterfly rash on the face) become evident. In fact, a 1994 study by E. C. Miguel and colleagues found that the "mental" symptoms of more than a quarter of SLE patients began either before or shortly after the onset of the disorder. Furthermore, the symptoms of most of these subjects—sadness, irritability, hopelessness, cognitive problems—are the types of symptoms most likely to be dismissed as functional ("all in the head") rather than biological. Consequently, many SLE patients are initially referred to psychiatrists. And a patient (particularly a woman) exhibiting "psychiatric" symptoms and complaining of vague aches and pains that can't be substantiated by a superficial exam and less-than-comprehensive lab tests is all too likely to be labeled as having "conversion disorder" (a fancy term for hysteria) and given psychotropic medications.

These drugs—in addition to masking symptoms of a worsening disorder—can severely compromise a patient's already abnormal brain function. In *Who Says You're Neurotic?* psychiatrist Abraham Twerski offers the example of a 42-year-old woman, "Claire," admitted to a hospital psychiatric unit after being labeled as severely depressed. Claire's behavior had become bizarre and uncharacteristic—for instance, she suddenly began using foul language, and ordered her mother and father out of her room when they came to visit. But Claire's psychiatrists, instead of investigating the causes of these symptoms, ascribed her personality changes to feelings of loneliness following the marriage of her son (who had previously lived at home with Claire). They prescribed antipsychotic drugs, which, far from helping their patient, caused her to become very confused and disoriented. Fortunately, before the drugs could cause lasting harm, a medical consultant was called in to evaluate Claire and diagnosed her as having SLE. Treatment with appropriate medications led to a complete remission of her behavioral abnormalities.

Another group of people who suffer from label-and-drug syndrome are more than a million "hyperactive" children being given Ritalin, an amphetamine-like medication. Ritalin can cause symptoms ranging from thought disorder to insomnia to cardiac arrhythmia. Studies indicate that it also stunts the growth of many children. There have been no long-term studies on Ritalin's safety, even though the drug has now been on the market for 30 years.

Many physicians believe that the known and potential risks associated with Ritalin are outweighed by its effectiveness as a treatment, but the scientific evidence proves them wrong. Long-term studies show that Ritalin doesn't "treat" hyperactivity; it simply masks symptoms that reappear as soon as the drug is stopped. Children taking Ritalin remain at high risk for school failure, delinquency, and severe behavioral problems that may plague them throughout their lives. As physician Leon Eisenberg, a professor at Harvard Medical School, recently noted, "There is just no evidence that over the long run, they [Ritalin and similar drugs] make a difference in the life of a child."

In short, years of Ritalin treatment leave patients no better off than they were before. Often, in fact, they are worse off, if their underlying brain dysfunctions are progressive.

A good example of this counterproductive drug treatment involved Charlie, a pale and rail-thin ten-year-old I once evaluated. Charlie suffered from violent mood swings: one minute he'd be giggling over nothing, and the next he'd be yelling obscenities or kicking his little sister. He couldn't control his temper at school, either; the day before I saw him, he'd reacted to another child's taunting on the playground by trying to run the boy down with his bike. Charlie had been in trouble for cursing at a teacher, throwing books in class, and breaking a window during a tantrum over an "F" on a math test. His teachers, who suspected that Charlie had "attention deficit disorder" or "conduct disorder," were asking that he be moved to a special education class.

Charlie's previous doctor had labeled him as hyperactive and had prescribed Ritalin for his moodiness, tantrums, and poor school performance. When Charlie's mother balked at taking the prescription, the doctor said, "You have two choices: give him Ritalin, or let him suffer." The guilt trip worked, and Charlie's mother filled the prescription—but she also wisely decided to get a second opinion.

When I examined Charlie I found many telltale signs of poor health, including his bad coloring, the ridges on his fingernails, and his frail build. My initial suspicions about what ailed Charlie grew stronger when his mother told me that one of Charlie's uncles and several of his cousins had diabetes. I performed physical, neurological, and biochemical evaluations, which revealed that Charlie had a very low level of glucose in his blood and that his insulin level was too high. This condition is often an early stage of diabetes, a disease characterized by the opposite symptoms: high blood sugar and low insulin. Either condition, if uncontrolled, can lead to mood swings, erratic behavior, and violent outbursts—the very symptoms "hyperactive" Charlie had exhibited.

After tests ruled out other metabolic problems, I diagnosed Charlie as having hyperinsulinism and placed him on an appropriate treatment program. Within a short time, his hyperactive behaviors cleared, his aggression and tantrums stopped, and his grades went up. Although Charlie's condition will require lifelong monitoring and management, it shouldn't prevent him from leading a perfectly normal life. But had Charlie's parents taken the first opinion they received, instead of seeking the true cause of their son's disorder, he would have taken a stimulant drug for years and his untreated prediabetic condition would have worsened. In addition, he might have found himself expelled from school, or even in trouble with the law, because of his violent behaviors.

Aaron, another boy I once saw, had taken Ritalin for more than two years after a fifteen-minute evaluation by a pediatrician. The drug made Aaron agitated, caused him to lose weight, and kept him awake at night. "He keeps begging me not to give it to him," his mother told me, "but the doctor says he needs it." But Aaron didn't need Ritalin at all; in fact, the drug was actually making his real medical problem worse.

When I questioned Aaron's mother, I learned that he was irritable and always tired. He was short for his age, and he had abnormal brain wave patterns (a sign of seizure activity). In addition, I learned that Aaron ate dirt and other nonfoods—a behavior called pica, which should lead a doctor to test for nutritional deficiencies (which can cause pica) and lead poisoning (which can result from the behavior).

Sure enough, further evaluation and studies revealed that Aaron suffered from iron-deficiency anemia, and that his lead levels were elevated. Ironically, the Ritalin prescribed by Aaron's previous doctor had—by reducing the boy's appetite—exacerbated his underlying nutritional deficiency. So, in this case, the "treatment" made the patient's condition worse.

Drug-Caused Illness

It's bad enough that psychotropic drugs don't treat brain dysfunction. Worse yet, however, they often create new and serious symptoms patients didn't have before "treatment." Drugs are alien substances that upset the natural chemical environment of neurons (the brain cells responsible for thought and behavior), causing these cells to compensate by altering their sensitivity or their own output of chemicals. These changes in turn affect surrounding cells, and eventually other areas of the brain, in a domino effect that disrupts the delicate and complex chemical balance of the brain. The more out of whack the brain's chemicals get, the more symptoms occur, and the harder it is to restore normal brain functioning.

Psychotropic drugs can be particularly dangerous for patients whose symptoms are traceable to toxic exposure. Consider, for instance, the patient whose brain dysfunction is caused by exposure to pesticides. The chemical "soup" surrounding and inside this patient's brain cells is already full of unnatural substances that are altering the transmissions between the cells. Adding toxic drugs to this mix—especially drugs that may react synergistically with the toxins already present—is, in effect, adding poisons to poisons.

Furthermore, drugs don't target a specific area of the brain that is malfunctioning. They affect *all* areas of the brain—and often other areas of the body as well. This shotgun approach frequently has catastrophic consequences. For instance:

- Many psychotropic drugs lower levels of dopamine, a chemical found in many areas of the brain, among them an area called the substantia nigra. Reducing dopamine levels in this tiny part of the brain can cause severe symptoms of parkinsonism, including uncontrollable shaking, muscle pain, listlessness, drooling, incontinence, a "zombie-like" expression, and despondency.
- Dopamine-blocking drugs can also disrupt the body's temperature-regulating mechanisms, leading to neuroleptic

malignant syndrome—a condition in which the body literally overheats. The disorder can cause coma and even death. Recent research by Richard D. Boyd suggests that the syndrome, which most physicians dismiss as rare, may in fact be responsible for many cases of unexplained death among mentally retarded and psychotic patients.

- Imipramine, an antidepressant prescribed to thousands of children for symptoms ranging from bed-wetting to aggression, can create hormonal imbalances in adolescents and adults. Men may develop breasts, and women who are not pregnant may begin producing breast milk.

- One side effect that is almost epidemic among patients taking certain types of neuroleptic drugs, including Haldol and Thorazine, is tardive dyskinesia (TD). This is a serious and sometimes permanent neurological disorder marked by abnormal involuntary muscle movements such as lip smacking, grimacing, and jerking. As many as 30 percent of patients taking neuroleptic drugs for extended periods develop TD. Patients with TD often have difficulty walking, sitting, breathing, talking, or eating normally, and they may develop dementia.

- A common side effect of Prozac and other neuroleptic drugs is akathisia, a syndrome whose symptoms include extreme restlessness, pacing or rocking from foot to foot, constant fidgeting, and sleeplessness. Patients who develop akathisia become irritable and aggressive, and may try to commit suicide or harm others.

- Prozac can also cause headaches, anxiety, dizziness, confusion, rashes, and swollen lymph nodes. Some users suffer from "Prozac syndrome," which includes muscle tremors, agitation, hot flashes, and nausea.

- Sexual dysfunction, once thought to be a rare effect of antidepressants, may in fact occur in more than a third of patients taking these drugs. One recent study, described in the *Journal of Clinical Psychiatry,* found that 43 percent of patients taking antidepressants reported sexual problems.

Another study, reported in the same journal, found that 34 percent of patients taking Prozac experienced diminished sexual desire or response.

- Studies have found that benzodiazepines—Valium, Xanax, and related drugs—impair memory. Psychiatrist Robert Gladstone has compared Xanax to "a big eraser" that wipes out patients' ability to pay attention, and psychiatrist Stuart Yudofsky says, "I think all benzodiazepines cause memory lapses, especially in the elderly." Benzodiazepines can also suppress breathing. In patients with lung disease or sleep apnea (a sleep disorder in which patients stop breathing many times during the night), benzodiazepine use can be life-threatening.

- Mark Riddle and colleagues report that at least four children have died from cardiac arrest caused by desipramine, an antidepressant used to treat conditions ranging from bed-wetting and school phobia to Tourette's syndrome and hyperactivity. And psychotropic drugs in general appear to dramatically increase the risk of fatal cardiac disorders: a recent study by Margaret Thorogood showed that young women taking psychotropic drugs were 17 times more likely than other young women to suffer heart attacks.

- Elderly patients taking psychotropic drugs greatly increase their risk of suffering hip fractures, an injury that often leads to rapid decline or even death. One reason is that many antipsychotic drugs cause hypotension (low blood pressure), which can lead to severe dizziness. Such drugs are particularly dangerous when combined with the blood pressure medications commonly prescribed for elderly patients.

- Transquilizers can cause incontinence, and antidepressants and antipsychotic drugs can cause urinary retention, particularly in patients with prostate problems.

- There is alarming, although preliminary, evidence that Prozac and other antidepressants may increase the growth rate of cancerous tumors. Canadian researcher Lorne Brandes gave Prozac and Elavil to animals with laboratory-induced cancers, feeding them doses equivalent to those used in humans. The drugs caused the animals' tumors to appear earlier and to grow to two or three times the size of those seen in control animals. A recent Japanese study found that Elavil speeded the growth of cancerous colon tumors in mice and rats, and German researchers have reported that melanomas—the deadliest form of cancer—grew faster in rodents given the antidepressant desipramine.

Human Guinea Pigs

One of the hazards of widespread prescribing of new drugs such as Prozac is that these drugs are marketed after short-term studies on limited populations. They almost inevitably have long-term side effects, but no one knows what these effects are until the drugs have been in use for years or decades. In effect, the millions of people using Prozac and other new drugs are human guinea pigs.

Most people taking new drugs don't realize this. Consumers tend to assume that all drugs are carefully tested on large groups of subjects, over long periods of time, and that any drugs found to be unsafe aren't approved. Unfortunately, that's not what happens. Most drug trials last weeks or months—not years—and involve only a few hundred patients. Side effects, even serious ones, aren't likely to be obvious until thousands of people have taken a drug over a number of years—circumstances that only occur once the drug is on the market.

Furthermore, drug companies—the very organizations that stand to profit handsomely if drugs are approved—fund much of the research used to determine whether new drugs are safe and effective. In the *New England Journal of Medicine,* physician Alan Hillman and colleagues describe how drug companies influence such research: "They fund projects with a high likelihood of producing favorable results. . . . They exclude products that may compare favorably with the sponsor's own. Sometimes, only favorable clinical data are released to investigators. . . . Negative studies may be terminated before they are ready for publication. . . . Corporate personnel may seek to control the content and use of the final report, including the decision to publish."

Here's an example of how this works. In 1981, Upjohn, a major drug company, introduced a new drug called Xanax. The goal: to corner the market on treating anxiety, which is big business for psychiatry. With numerous other drugs already being prescribed for anxiety, Upjohn had to produce some pretty impressive statistics about Xanax in order to woo doctors.

Upjohn spent a fortune on studies carefully tailored to produce exactly the desired results. The biggest of these was the "Cross-National Panic Study" conducted in different cities around the world. Glowing reports on the study results were published in psychiatric journals.

There was only one problem: the study *didn't prove that Xanax was particularly effective*. Phase One of the study did show that after four weeks, 50 percent of patients taking Xanax had no panic attacks, compared to 28 percent of the patients taking placebos (fake pills). That is what Upjohn boasted about in its advertising. What Upjohn didn't mention, however, was that after eight weeks, at the end of the study, *patients taking Xanax were having as many panic attacks as those on the placebo*. Even more importantly, Upjohn didn't mention the fact that the "rebound" effect that occurred when patients stopped taking Xanax was devastating in many cases. Canadian researchers involved in the Cross-National Panic Study reported that both Xanax and placebo groups were averaging about two panic attacks a week when the study ended. But the patients who took Xanax for eight weeks and then went off the drug were suffering nearly *seven attacks a week* after two weeks of withdrawal—while those who stopped taking the placebo continued to suffer only about two attacks a week. In addition, the Cross-National Panic Study showed that imipramine, a drug already on the market, was as effective (or, from another point of view, as ineffective) as Xanax. Yet the "data" from this study, published in major medical journals and promoted in glossy ads, were enough to convince doctors to write millions of prescriptions for Xanax, quickly making it one of America's most popular psychotropic drugs.

Lest you think this was a one-time occurrence, consider Upjohn's marketing of Halcion, a tranquilizer that caused severe side effects in many patients. The U.S. Food and Drug Administration (FDA), which investigated Upjohn's research and marketing of the drug, charged that the company "engaged in an ongoing pattern of misconduct" to conceal the drug's dangers. According to the FDA's investigators, Upjohn sought approval of the drug at one-milligram doses, even though research indicated this was a dangerously high dose; withheld from the FDA data of severe adverse reactions to Halcion; and sought approval for long-term prescribing of the drug, "even though available evidence indicated that long-term use was both dangerous and medically untenable."

"Drug risks will always be unacceptably high," consumer activist Charles Medawar writes in *Power and Dependence*, "so long as the industry tends to pour money into demonstrating product benefits, while pouring cold water on allegations of risk—calling on quite different standards of investigation and proof in each case." Until a better system for drug testing is established, dangerous drugs will continue to gain approval and be administered to millions of unsuspecting patients.

Previous generations of Americans have learned the hard way about the dangers of being guinea pigs for poorly tested drugs. In the early 1900s, millions of people took bromides, prescribed as a cure for everything from battlefield anxiety to masturbation. Bromides were given to pregnant women for "nerves," to children for "overactivity," and to just about anybody who couldn't sleep well at night. By 1930, four out of every ten prescriptions written by doctors were for drugs containing bromides. It took doctors nearly half a century to recognize (and admit) that bromides were terribly toxic, and that thousands of Americans were suffering from anxiety, dementia, or schizophrenia-like symptoms brought on entirely by "bromide intoxication." By then, many of their patients were in mental institutions. Ironically, most doctors had considered the early symptoms of bromide poisoning—restlessness, disorientation, paranoia, hallucinations, and apprehension—to be signs that a patient needed *more* bromides, and had medicated many of these patients into chronic insanity!

As bromides gradually fell out of favor, the drug companies replaced them with barbiturates—"minor" tranquilizers billed as "absolutely safe and without toxic effects." It took nearly 50 years for physicians to realize that these drugs could be more addictive than morphine. Even after they did, it took another decade or so for barbiturates to fall totally out of favor. In the meantime, thousands of people who took barbiturates wound up addicted and lost their jobs and families.

Around this time, another barbiturate-like drug was introduced as a mild tranquilizer suitable even for pregnant women. (In fact, much of the drug's promotion was specifically aimed at pregnant women.) You may remember the drug's name: thalidomide. Approximately ten thousand women who took thalidomide gave birth to children who were missing arms and legs or were otherwise seriously deformed.

Then came Librium, Valium, Xanax, and the other benzodiazepine drugs that replaced the barbiturates. Again, drug companies and doctors described these drugs as safe—and, again, they were wrong. We know now that children whose mothers took Valium and similar drugs while pregnant have an increased risk of hyperactivity and learning disabilities. We know that Halcion, a sleeping pill heralded as a wonder drug in the mid-1980s, caused terrible insomnia, hostility, paranoia, or amnesia in hundreds of patients. And we know that all of the minor tranquilizers so popular in the 1980s and early 1990s are much more addictive than initially thought.

In short, virtually every "safe" or "harmless" psychotropic drug introduced on the market was later found to have serious or even fatal side effects. The long-term effects of newer drugs are quite likely to be just as bad—and by the time we learn what they are, it will be too late for many of the people taking them. Many psychiatrists justify the use of such dangerous drugs by analyzing the drugs' "risk–benefit ratio"—in other words, by comparing the potential side effects of drugs to their potential benefits. But even assuming that these comparisons are accurate—which they usually aren't, because studies tend to inflate benefits and underestimate risks—why take *any* risk in cases where brain dysfunction can be diagnosed and treated *without* psychotropic drugs?

It's human nature to get excited about a new "miracle drug," especially if the manufacturer claims it can cure a frightening or crippling disorder. But all drugs are double-edged swords. Even the best drugs cause side effects, and the worst drugs—including most psychotropic drugs—can cause severe adverse reactions or even death. Drug companies play up the beneficial aspects of their products while downplaying their adverse effects (or, in many cases, neglecting to warn patients about them at all). And far too few physicians remember that the purpose of prescriptions is to allow physicians to *protect patients from taking drugs that are dangerous or inappropriate.* The prescription pad should be a means of limiting drug misuse, not fostering it.

One way to learn about the side effects of psychotropic drugs is to consult the *Physician's Desk Reference* (PDR). Compiled by drug companies and distributed to physicians, the PDR lists the known side effects of most commonly prescribed drugs. Although most people think of the PDR as a reference manual, it's actually a device to reduce drug companies' legal liability: by issuing a public listing of the known toxic effects of their products, the companies can claim to have informed consumers about these effects (even though few physicians pass the PDR information on to their patients).

You'll certainly learn more about the negative effects of psychotropic drugs from the PDR than from DSM-IV, which barely mentions the topic of iatrogenic (physician-caused) illness, even though a large percentage of patients experience serious symptoms (including brain dysfunction) caused partly or entirely by the medications prescribed for them by their physicians.

Can Psychotropic Drugs Make You Crazy?

Besides the unpleasant side effects already noted, there are other reasons not to take psychotropic drugs. A key reason is that these drugs, designed to reduce behavioral symptoms, often *cause* them.

- Xanax can cause sadness, confusion, manic symptoms, hostility, paranoia, increased agitation, and self-mutilation. According to one study, eight of 80 patients given Xanax became angry, extremely hostile, or violent. One patient in this group, a woman who had never been violent before, began screaming wildly, and at one point held a steak knife to her mother's throat.
- Valium can cause confusion, rage reactions, and hallucinations. (John Hinckley, Jr., who attempted to assassinate President Reagan, apparently was under the influence of Valium on the day of the attack.)
- Thorazine can cause confusion, hallucinations, disorientation, memory loss, and dementia.
- Lithium can cause dementia and memory impairment.
- Monoamine oxidase inhibitors (a class of antidepressants) can cause mania, confusion, memory loss, irritability, sleeplessness, and agitation.
- Ritalin has been blamed for several murders committed by children who reacted violently to the drug.
- Halcion, a sleeping pill that has been banned in Britain, is still available in the United States. Author Philip Roth plunged into a suicidal depression after being given the drug while recuperating from minor knee surgery. And author William Styron, who took Halcion when he experienced anxiety before an operation, said later, in an article in *The Nation*, that he became "all but totally consumed by thoughts of suicide that were like a form of lust. Somehow I managed to get through my classroom duties, but my mind was never free of exquisite pain, a pain that had but one solution—self-extinction." When he wrote of his experiences,

Styron says, he was "stunned" by the stacks of mail he received from former Halcion users describing the homicidal or suicidal urges they experienced while taking the drug.

My first experience with brain dysfunction caused by psychotropic drugs involved a young, healthy, and very capable surgical nurse (I'll call her "Nurse M") with whom I'd worked during my neurosurgical residency. Shortly after I began my psychiatric residency, Nurse M was admitted to the hospital with a label of acute schizophrenia, and I happened to be assigned to her case.

I knew Nurse M's problem was serious when I first saw her in the emergency room. When I said hello to her, Nurse M—who had scrubbed with me on dozens of surgeries, eaten lunch with me in the hospital cafeteria, and said "Hi" to me in the hallways every day for months—stared at me blankly as if she'd never seen me before. In addition, she wasn't the least bit embarrassed to have me examine her. (Most hospital employees are mortified when they wind up being patients themselves.) This usually neat-as-a-pin young woman was a mess: her hair was a rat's nest, her mascara was smeared under her eyes, and her clothes looked like they hadn't been changed for days. It wasn't hard to determine that Nurse M indeed had lost touch with reality. I was also able to determine, however, that she wasn't "schizophrenic."

I gained several important clues about Nurse M's real disorder from her personal and medical history. For instance, she was pregnant, had been having difficulty sleeping, and was taking barbiturates she had obtained surreptitiously from the hospital. (In those days, it was considered "normal" to take barbiturates for minor sleeping problems, even during pregnancy.)

Pregnancy and barbiturates both can trigger symptoms of acute intermittent porphyria in people who carry the dominant gene for this disorder (which interferes with the breakdown of body chemicals called porphyrins, causing them to accumulate in toxic amounts). Most people have no idea that they carry the gene for porphyria until biological or environmental stresses—

drugs, starvation, changes in sex hormones, or infections—trigger symptoms such as abdominal pain, insomnia, nervousness, confusion, hallucinations, and seizures. Although porphyria's most famous victim was the "Mad King," George III of England, whose attacks of porphyria eventually led to his removal from the throne, the disease strikes women more often than men.

The lab tests I ordered for Nurse M showed the presence of elevated levels of porphyrins in her urine and blood. (The urine is often a distinctive port-wine color in porphyria patients.) Once the diagnosis was established, on the basis of a detailed history and comprehensive examination, I was able to manage Nurse M's condition by prescribing an anticonvulsant for use during acute episodes and counseling her about the factors, such as barbiturate use, that bring on attacks. Nurse M was able to return to nursing and subsequently moved to another state, where she gave birth to a perfectly normal baby girl. Her obstetrician, warned about her porphyria, was careful not to administer any drugs that would trigger an attack. I received a thank-you note from her shortly afterward, along with a photo of her baby.

Luckily for Nurse M, I wasn't a practitioner of DSM medicine. Otherwise, I might have labeled her as "schizophrenic" and continued treating her with medications similar to the barbiturates she'd been taking—in effect, making her permanently brain-damaged due to elevated porphyrins.

Nurse M suffered from a fairly rare disorder that increased her risk of drug-induced brain dysfunction, but psychotropic drugs can cause similar symptoms in *anyone*. Furthermore, symptoms can occur after a prolonged period of seemingly symptom-free drug use, and they can be triggered by combining psychotropic drugs with relatively innocuous over-the-counter medications.

Given the potential of psychotropic drugs to create brain dysfunction, it's particularly frightening that they are increasingly being prescribed for people who have no symptoms of psychiatric disorder at all. Prozac, for instance, is currently prescribed for millions of healthy people seeking "designer personalities"—even though it is a powerful drug whose long-term consequences are completely unknown. (The drug's use as a personality pill is so widespread that its manufacturer, Eli Lilly, took the unusual step of criticizing "the unprecedented amount of media attention" Prozac is receiving, and discouraging physicians from prescribing it unless "a clear medical need exists." The warning, however, seems to have had little effect on some in the psychiatric community.)

Similarly, Ritalin, an amphetamine-like drug that many physicians concede has no long-term beneficial effects, is now prescribed for more than one million American schoolchildren, most of whom have no pathological symptoms but are merely "squirmy." And tricyclic antidepressants, which can cause hallucinations, convulsions, and cardiac arrest, are routinely prescribed for adolescents undergoing the admittedly painful, but totally normal, process of growing up.

The main culprit responsible for this medication of normal children and adults is the DSM. The symptoms listed under each DSM label are so vague and arbitrary that a drug-oriented physician can stretch the definitions to fit almost any patient. For example, take one more look at the DSM list of symptoms for "hyperactivity," first introduced in Chapter 1:

1. Often fidgets with hands or feet or squirms in seat.
2. Often leaves seat in classroom or in other situations in which remaining seated in expected.
3. Often runs about or climbs excessively in situations in which it is inappropriate (in adolescents or adults, may be limited to subjective feelings of restlessness).
4. Often has difficulty playing or engaging in leisure activities quietly.
5. Is often "on the go" or often acts as if "driven by a motor."
6. Often talks excessively.
7. Often blurts out answers before questions have been completed.
8. Often has difficulty awaiting turn.
9. Often interrupts or intrudes on others (e.g., butts into conversations or games).

Without exaggerating a bit, I can say that this list describes virtually every child ever born. In fact, I would worry about a child who *didn't* exhibit five or six of these symptoms. Presumably, the DSM relies on psychiatrists to use their clinical judgment as to the severity of symptoms. But a DSM-oriented psychiatrist, faced with a parent who has read about the "wonder drug" Ritalin and pressured by teachers who want the disruptive child "calmed down," is under substantial pressure to prescribe the drug to a child exhibiting symptoms that are well within the range of normality. And the psychiatrist would be going by the book: after all, hyperactivity is the *accepted DSM label* for a child with six or more of the symptoms on the list, and Ritalin is the *accepted treatment* for a DSM label of "hyperactivity."

Similarly, the symptoms required for a DSM label of "anxiety disorder" or "depression" are vague enough to include many people experiencing normal reactions to life. If your best friend dies, it's normal and healthy to grieve—sometimes for a long time. If you recover from a life-threatening illness, or survive a war, it's normal to feel anxious or depersonalized, and to experience fears of death. But it's easy for a psychiatrist to stretch such normal responses to fit the DSM definitions of "mental illness," and treat them with drugs. Often this is done with the best of intentions—after all, few of us can stand to watch another human endure prolonged suffering. But suffering is an integral part of the human experience. Much like overprotective parents who refuse to let their children ride bikes or play baseball because they might get hurt, psychiatrists who offer patients pills in an attempt to protect them from the hard knocks of life are doing them no service.

Breaking Our Oath

A good physician uses drug therapies only after careful diagnostic procedures have ruled out all other avenues. Physicians who skip the work of making an accurate diagnosis, and cavalierly prescribe dangerous psychotropic drugs based solely on labels picked out of the DSM, are violating one of the most basic principles of medicine: *to do no harm*. And physicians who prescribe drugs to perfectly normal, healthy patients looking for a magic pill to make them more popular, or less sensitive to life's ups and downs, are even more misguided: they are actually *creating* brain dysfunction where none existed, and stunting their patients' emotional growth as well. Even physicians who prescribe psychotropic drugs for the kindly reason of helping patients through grief or trauma are doing harm rather than good because they are teaching their patients that all bad feelings must be drugged away.

As Captain Joseph Pursch, the Navy doctor whom former First Lady Betty Ford credits for her recovery from drug addiction, told the authors of *The Tranquilizing of America*, "If you come to me with an emotional problem, you want help. I really can't help you by giving you a pill. The act of giving you a pill reduces your humanness. If I give you a pill, I reinforce all the negative forces in you. By giving you a tranquilizer prescription for an emotional problem, I am saying that you are inadequate, that your humanness does not count, and that you need a pill to live. By giving you a pill, I diminish you."

A patient's health is his or her most prized possession. To prescribe medicines known to cause grave risk to a patient's health, and known to have few beneficial effects, is a perversion of the physician's duty and a violation of the Hippocratic Oath. To prescribe such drugs as a means of helping patients shirk responsibility or avoid life's tough knocks is simply unconscionable. These practices should be strongly condemned—not actively encouraged—by the American Psychiatric Association.

CHAPTER 4

Prescription Junkies

I told my doctor I was afraid of addiction. She was emphatic. "Look, these are harmless drugs. As long as you follow my prescription you have no need to worry about becoming an addict."

Max Ricketts, author of The Great Anxiety Escape,
describing the beginnings of his addiction to benzodiazepines

A FEW YEARS AGO, I EVALUATED MRS. LI, A SMALL, SAD, middle-aged Chinese woman. "Can you help me?," she asked haltingly, through her interpreter. I could, indeed, I replied after I'd made a diagnosis—but first we had to undo the "help" other psychiatrists had given her.

Shortly after arriving in the United States from Beijing, Mrs. Li was crossing a busy street in a California city when she was struck and knocked down by a truck driven by a city maintenance worker. At the time I saw her, she was suing the city for nearly a million dollars, claiming that the accident "did something terrible to my mind." The city, in turn, was accusing her of faking her problems. I found, upon examining her, that Mrs. Li's symptoms were real enough—but they had nothing to do with the accident, and a great deal to do with DSM nondiagnosis and irresponsible drug prescribing.

Mrs. Li appeared at my office dressed in a Mandarin top and pants, and smelling strongly of the sweet odor of incense. She was unkempt, had puffy eyes and a sallow, unhealthy skin color, and looked as though she hadn't changed her clothes in several days. The interpreter translated Mrs. Li's list of symptoms: insomnia, sadness, and, above all, overwhelming fatigue. Our interview was punctuated by Mrs. Li's frequent and copious tears.

75

Mrs. Li told me she was so exhausted that she spent most of her days on the couch watching television. "I don't visit my friends any more," she said, "because I don't want them to see what's happened to me. I sent my family in China some pictures of me, and they asked what made me grow old so fast." In fluent Mandarin, slowly translated into English by her companion, Mrs. Li told me she suffered from chronic, debilitating headaches, sometimes heard voices, and wept and laughed uncontrollably. In addition, she'd suffered a substantial hearing loss and frequently heard a ringing in her ears.

Mrs. Li had been "diagnosed" by several psychiatrists as having posttraumatic stress disorder, resulting from her accident. They had prescribed Xanax, Valium, Halcion, and imipramine. (When these didn't work, Mrs. Li supplemented them with an arsenal of Chinese herbal remedies, which proved equally ineffective.) By the time I saw Mrs. Li, she'd been a semi-invalid for over a year and was well on her way to becoming addicted to her prescription drugs.

Mrs. Li's underlying disorder, it turned out, was seronegative syphilis. Her ear disturbances and "mental" symptoms were traceable to this infection, which I treated with antibiotics. But that didn't end her troubles, because she had a second problem: drug dependency.

Unfortunately, prescription drug addiction is a problem I see all too often. Many patients, although cured of their original brain dysfunction, still face the ordeal of giving up drugs on which they've become hooked. Although the motives of the psychiatrists who prescribed these drugs were the best—to ease the pain and suffering of patients—the consequences of their unchecked prescribing of addictive drugs have been disastrous.

Progress in Psychiatry: From Cocaine to Valium

Psychiatry's love affair with potentially addictive drugs stretches back to Freud and his contemporaries. In fact, one of the most famous cases ever presented by Sigmund Freud—that of "Anna O.," who was actually treated by Josef Breuer—was notable not because Breuer cured her (she later spent almost two years in an asylum), but because she was one of modern psychiatry's first recorded cases of iatrogenic (doctor-caused) drug addiction. In addition to psychoanalyzing her, Breuer gave her massive quantities of chloral hydrate, and her later doctors administered doses of morphine ten times higher than the amounts currently used for postoperative patients.

Meanwhile, Freud himself was spreading the word about a new wonder drug, telling friends and patients that "the psychic effect of [the drug] consists of exhilaration and lasting euphoria which does not differ from normal euphoria of a healthy person," and that "absolutely no craving for further use . . . appears after the first or repeated taking." The drug? Cocaine.

Freud and Breuer may have been the first mental health professionals to promote drugs leading to abuse and addiction, but they certainly weren't the last. In the 1960s, psychologist Timothy Leary called on Americans to "open our minds" by trying LSD. As late as 1985, *The Comprehensive Textbook of Psychiatry* claimed that cocaine, "if used moderately and occasionally, . . . creates no serious problems." And the hallucinogenic drug Ecstasy, which permanently damages brain cells and has caused hundreds of deaths due to cardiac dysfunction or cerebral hemorrhage, was frequently recommended to patients by psychotherapists during the 1970s and early 1980s as a means of facilitating insight-oriented therapy, despite early recognition of its lethal effects.

Today, psychiatrists know that cocaine, Ecstasy, and LSD are dangerous, and society outlaws these drugs. Instead, many psychiatrists prescribe Valium, Xanax, Ritalin, and related drugs. In fact, these drugs are often the *only* treatment—other than psychotherapy—recommended by DSM-oriented psychiatrists. But is the rationale of these psychiatrists any better than Freud's or Timothy Leary's? And are these drugs any better than the street drugs we campaign against? The answer, usually, is no.

DSM's label-and-drug approach teaches both physicians and patients that a successful office visit ends with a prescription in the patient's hand. In many cases, however, there is little difference between the drug being prescribed and the drugs being sold on street corners. Like illegal drugs, prescription psychotropic drugs can cause hallucinations, paranoia, and aggression. And like illegal drugs, psychotropic drugs frequently cause outright addiction.

Benzodiazepines, for instance—Librium, Valium, Xanax, and related drugs—are considered to be minor tranquilizers, and are often given to patients who have only mild symptoms of distress or anxiety. They are, as one doctor put it, "the holy water of psychiatry." At the height of these drugs' popularity, in the early 1980s, more than one in every ten Americans was taking them—usually for minor stress or sleeping problems. Although that number has dropped, millions of Americans still take benzodiazepines each year—many of them, according to a *Consumer Reports* series on the drugs, "people who have no psychiatric diagnosis at all." (It's no surprise that the first benzodiazepine introduced on the market, in the 1960s, was promoted with the advertising slogan, "Whatever the diagnosis . . . Librium.")

Yet a recent research review by Norman Miller and Mark Gold, in *The American Journal of Drug and Alcohol Abuse,* concludes that "dependence [on benzodiazepines] occurs rapidly, within a few weeks, perhaps days," and that withdrawal from the drugs causes dozens of severe symptoms ranging from intense anxiety and panic attacks to depression, hallucinations, shortness of breath, vomiting, headaches, and paranoid delusions. In addition, withdrawal from benzodiazepines often causes a "rebound" effect: the symptoms the patient experienced before taking the drug recur, but in a much more severe form. (Ironically, psychiatrists often assume this means that the patient still "needs" the drugs—an assumption that results in another prescription.) Max Ricketts, a former State Department official whose physicians prescribed benzodiazepines for anxiety attacks, describes in *The Great Anxiety Escape* how painful withdrawal from these drugs can be:

Odors made me nauseated. My foot did not know where it would step when I tried to walk. The slightest sound was an explosion in my ears. Every nerve ending was screaming in pain. Yet I could not even cry. The instinctive will to survive was overwhelmed by the fear of living in this unreal, uncontrollable hell . . . I wanted to die, but I couldn't organize my thoughts enough to do it.

Another patient who became addicted to Valium told his story to Eve Bargmann, M.D. and her colleagues, in *Stopping Valium:*

I stopped, and for the first couple of weeks it was terror; multiple muscle contractions. I think one of the best descriptions I have heard is if somebody pours kerosene over your skin and then every so often they touch a torch to it. . . . I became very paranoid; everybody was out to get me and nobody was a friend any longer. . . . I became so uptight that I could not sleep; I could not eat.

Such reactions aren't rare; in fact, three thousand Britons sued the drug firms of Wyeth and Hoffmann-La Roche in 1991, charging that they had become addicted to either Valium or Ativan (benzodiazepines commonly prescribed for anxiety) after receiving inadequate warning about the drugs' addictive potential. And when Ricketts wrote an article in a Manila newspaper describing his ordeal (which led to an unsuccessful suicide attempt before he recovered), hundreds of readers came forward to describe their own addiction to benzodiazepines. It has become increasingly clear that drug companies' initial claims that these drugs weren't addictive, except when given to alcoholics and others with "addictive personalities," were false. Regarding benzodiazepine addiction, as one doctor put it, there is no "we" and "they"—everyone is equally at risk.

Research studies clearly show that benzodiazepines—particularly Xanax, currently one of America's most popular drugs—are as addictive as many "hard core" street drugs. In one study, Karl Rickels and his colleagues at the University of Pennsylvania tried to wean 47 patients, who'd been taking benzodiazepines for a year or more, off the drugs. Fifty-seven percent of the patients taking Xanax or chemically similar benzodiazepines were unable to stop, and 27 percent of the patients taking Valium and similar drugs found that they couldn't quit. A Canadian study found that two-thirds of long-term Xanax users had tried to stop using the drug but had failed.

"If you told your doctor that you were anxious and he or she recommended that you treat it by drinking a pint of whiskey a day for the next six months, you would probably be shocked," Bargmann says. "Yet valium and all benzodiazepines, like alcohol, are addicting drugs—and a [single] prescription, especially one with refills, may give you enough to result in addiction."

The tragedy of benzodiazepine dependence is that it's unnecessary. I've found, in my own practice, that the vast majority of anxiety attacks can be cured by diagnosing their underlying causes—which can include poor diet, excessive caffeine, hyperventilation, and cardiac problems. Conversely, there's little evidence that the drugs given to combat anxiety actually benefit patients. W. K. Zung and colleagues, who compared tranquilizers to sugar pills, found that the placebos worked just as well. In another study, J. Catalan and fellow researchers divided 90 patients with anxiety into two groups: one group took benzodiazepines, and the other received therapy involving simple "listening, explanation, advice, and reassurance." The two treatments were equally effective, and patients actually preferred the latter approach.

Benzodiazepines account for most cases of addiction to psychiatric drugs, but they aren't the only drugs that can cause dependency. A study by Steven Dilsaver, in *International Clinical Psychopharmacology,* reported that more than half of patients taking antidepressants have difficulty cutting back on their dosage, and experience symptoms such as anxiety, panic, and irrationality. Reports of addiction to monoamine oxidase inhibitors, one form of antidepressants, are beginning to trickle in. Ritalin, which mimics the effects of amphetamines when taken in high doses, and pemoline, another drug prescribed for hyperactivity, can also be addictive.

Amazingly, few physicians adequately warn their patients about the risks of drug dependence and addiction. Typical is the case of actress Winona Ryder, who became dependent on tranquilizers prescribed for insomnia after her doctor reassured her that "you can eat them like candy."

Many cases of addiction occur in patients receiving multiple prescriptions written by different doctors. This is a common problem among the elderly, who often become—in the words of Charles Inlander—"prescription junkies." In *Worst Pills/Best Pills*, Sidney Wolfe, M.D., and colleagues charge that "the majority of . . . older adults in this country who regularly use these pills have become addicted to benzodiazepine tranquilizers and sleeping pills, thanks to their doctors and the drug industry."

Even drugs that do not appear to cause overt physical symptoms often become a crutch, because they provide a means of hiding from real-life problems. In *The Brain has a Mind of its Own*, neurologist and author Richard Restak voices concern that Prozac and similar drugs "will lead to the same behavioral patterns of every other mood- and behavior-altering drug: withdrawal, self-absorption, a lack of concern about anything other than what's happening inside the user's head." Restak fears that such drugs will lead users to conclude that "if the world isn't behaving as you believe that it should, and you feel good while taking your own special drug, then say no to the world rather than to the drug."

Are We "Pushing" Legal Drugs?

The similarities between street drug abuse and psychotropic prescription drug use are disturbing. Both types of drugs are toxic. Both can cause psychosis, damage the brain and other organs, and even cause death. *And neither type of mind-altering drugs, legal or illegal, treats disease.* It's important to recognize that the only significant difference between many prescription psychotropic drugs and street drugs such as "speed" and "downers" is that prescription drugs are legal.

Furthermore, the reasons addicts give for using street drugs sound much like the reasons some psychiatrists give for prescribing psychotropic drugs. Ask a cocaine user why he or she takes the drug, and you'll hear, "It makes me feel like I can accomplish anything. It give me confidence. I can't function without it. It makes me feel better." Ask some psychiatrists why they prescribe benzodiazepines or Prozac for patients with mild anxiety or distress—or sometimes with no symptoms at all—and you'll hear, "It makes them feel better." Or, "They can't function without it." Or, "It gives them confidence. It makes them feel like they can accomplish their goals." Psychiatrists, unlike illegal drug pushers, believe they are doing their clients a service—but good intentions aren't enough when the end result is dependency or addiction.

If the comparison between prescription drugs such as Valium and street drugs such as cocaine sounds far-fetched, consider the story of an airline stewardess named Carol. Her experience, related by Richard Hughes and Robert Brewin in *The Tranquilizing of America,* is a typical one. Carol was first prescribed Librium, and later Valium, when she told her doctor that she loved her new job, but was having a little trouble adjusting to the stress and the frequent changes in time zones. "Take these, dear, whenever you feel a bit anxious or under stress," her doctor said.

"The Valium did wonders for me, at least for a while," she told Hughes and Brewin. "One pill three or four times a day kept me in that mellow mood. . . . Then it became two Valiums, then three, and . . . I don't know how many I was taking at a time or how many times a day I was taking them toward the end." Carol began dropping passengers' trays during her flights. She experienced blackouts and fell frequently. Other doctors wrote her prescriptions for Tuinal (a barbiturate) and Tofranil (an antidepressant). She became paranoid and reclusive, and started missing flights. Her life, she said, "withered away to almost nothing, just the television set, the pills, and me." She finally overdosed on the drugs, and nearly died.

To anyone who has worked with cocaine addicts, alcoholics, or heroin junkies, Carol's story sounds all too familiar: escalating dosages, more and more drugs, blackouts, paranoia, and a life that revolves around the next "fix." The only major difference between Carol and street-corner junkies is that her drugs were legal.

Psychiatrists who really care about their patients—and I believe the overwhelming majority of them do—need to think about such cases (which aren't as rare as drug companies would like you to believe), and to take a hard look at what they're doing to patients when they prescribe mind-altering drugs. They can start by considering this test, entitled "Five Questions to Determine Whether Drug Use Is Appropriate or Constitutes Abuse," presented recently in the *American Family Physician* by Eric Voth and colleagues. Intended to help general practitioners spot patients who are abusing drugs, the test is equally useful for spotting "prescription pad abuse." The authors say that "one to five negative responses usually indicate inappropriate or nonmedical use." In my opinion, here's how the mind-altering drugs that psychiatrists commonly prescribe stack up.

1. *Is the drug used for a legitimate medical purpose?*

Usually not, because psychotropic drugs mask symptoms rather than treating the cause of a disorder. Furthermore, they are generally prescribed for patients who have been tagged with a DSM label after receiving little or no medical evaluation—the basis for any legitimate medical treatment. And they are too frequently given to patients with DSM labels such as "phase of life problem" or "dysthymia" (a term that translates to "a mild case of the blahs")—people with no real medical problems at all. In addition, many psychiatric drugs don't do what they promise to do. Benzodiazepines, for instance, appear to be ineffective after a few weeks—yet they're generally prescribed for long-term use.

2. *Does the drug improve the quality of the patient's life?*

Usually not, because the short-term relief psychiatric drugs provide is generally outweighed by their long-term effects—including addiction, severe sleep disturbance, sexual problems, and profound neurological dysfunction. Furthermore, patients' underlying disorders are left untreated and generally grow worse. And patients who become addicted frequently suffer from terrible guilt, because of the stigma society attaches to addiction—even when it occurs in innocent victims of improperly prescribed medications.

3. *Is the physician helping the patient maintain control over use of the drug?*

Almost never. Psychiatric drugs are generally prescribed for long-term use, with little physician supervision, thus maximizing the chance of addiction and reducing the patient's control over drug use. Most patients have little contact with their doctors after a drug is prescribed, except for quick visits at prescription-renewal time. These appointments, which psychiatrists sincerely think of as "evaluations," usually are quick in-and-out visits for which the psychiatrist collects $50 to $100 merely for writing a prescription refill.

4. *Is the use of the drug legal and uncomplicated by illegal drug use?*

Not always. The original prescription is of course legal, but a large number of prescription drug users develop addictions that expand into illegal drug use. A patient given a six-month prescription of Valium or Xanax, for instance, is at high risk of becoming addicted, and is quite likely to turn to street drugs in desperation when the prescription runs out. And many patients mix prescription psychiatric drugs with alcohol—a legal but potentially lethal combination.

5. *Is the pattern of use one of appropriate medicinal doses or is it one of intoxicating doses?*

"Intoxication" is defined in DSM-IV as "disturbances of perception, wakefulness, attention, thinking, judgment, psychomotor behavior, and interpersonal behavior" that are due to the effects of an intoxicating substance on the nervous system, and that "generally [place] the individual at significant risk for adverse effects (e.g., accidents, general medical complications, disruption in social and family relationships, vocational or financial difficulties, legal problems)." Thus, the nursing home patient drugged into a stupor on Stelazine could be considered "intoxicated." So could the patient who suffers a rage reaction while taking Xanax, or the employee who can't function on the job because of side effects of Valium, or the elderly patient who becomes disoriented, falls, and breaks a hip while taking Haldol. So could the 23,000 patients who had complained to the FDA, by 1992, that they had suffered adverse reactions to Prozac—including delirium, hallucinations, convulsions, violent hostility and aggression, psychosis, and suicidal thoughts.

Note that, according to this test, psychiatrists prescribing mind-altering drugs frequently fail to meet *any* of the criteria for appropriate drug administration!

Given the grim history of psychoactive "wonder drugs" that turned out to be societal problems, one would expect the psychiatric profession to err on the side of caution in prescribing potentially addictive medications—especially when they appear to do so little good. As I've noted, the track record of psychotropic drugs is poor: cocaine turned out to be addictive, so psychiatrists (after experimenting with chloral hydrate, which also proved to be addictive) turned to bromides. Bromides caused psychosis, so doctors started prescribing barbiturates. Barbiturates turned out to be addictive and often deadly, so benzodiazepines came into favor. Benzodiazepines caused addiction and rage reactions. Now psychiatrists are prescribing Prozac, saying—yet again—that it's "perfectly safe." The historical lesson to be learned here is not a comforting one.

It's important to remember, however, that a number of DSM-oriented psychiatrists have, to a large degree, abandoned the science of differential diagnosis, and thus consider most psychiatric illnesses "incurable." This leaves them with only two weapons: psychotherapy and drugs. It's not surprising that they're among the first to leap on each new drug bandwagon; like long-ago doctors who recommended bleeding for every ailment, they have little else to offer their patients.

As I've noted, psychiatry has weaned itself away from some of the drugs most likely to cause addiction or illegal drug use. Barbiturates, popular decades ago, are no longer considered appropriate, and although benzodiazepines are still prescribed for millions of patients every year, their use is gradually declining. Unfortunately, however, the use of LSD, Ecstasy and other hallucinogenic drugs in psychotherapy appears to be making a comeback; UCLA is testing Ecstasy "in anticipation of therapeutic applications," and the University of Miami is testing the hallucinogenic plant extract ibogaine. A recent article in the *Journal of Nervous and Mental Disease,* by psychiatrist Rick Strassman, claims that "the renewal of human hallucinogen research is encouraging" and that "courses of therapy utilizing adjunctive, high-dose, hallucinogen-assisted sessions should be considered"—particularly in light of the fact that "economic constraints create increasing pressure for cost-effective medical psychotherapy." The idea that drugs known to create hallucinations, behavioral disturbances, flashbacks, and outright psychosis can be beneficial in treating brain dysfunction—and "cost-effective" as well—is, to say the least, misguided.

I'm relatively confident that the public (if not the psychiatric profession) will reject a return to "treatment" with LSD and other psychedelic drugs, because the dangers of these drugs are far too well known. In addition, I think the use of benzodiazepines will continue to drop as people become more aware of their addictive potential. However, I have concerns about a new generation of drugs that are being sold to the public as "safe."

An Unanswered Question: Is Prozac Addictive?

The most popular psychotropic drug to hit the market in recent years is the antidepressant Prozac, currently being prescribed for a long list of DSM labels including depression, obsessive-compulsive disorder, dysthymic disorder, avoidant personality disorder, histrionic personality disorder, dependent personality disorder, and adjustment disorder. One of the drug's biggest selling points, according to many psychiatrists, is that it's not addictive. Unfortunately, the real truth, according to the *Physician's Desk Reference,* is that "Prozac has not been systematically studied, in animals or humans, for its potential for abuse, tolerance, or physical dependence," and that "it is not possible to predict on the basis of . . . limited experience the extent to which [Prozac] will be misused, diverted, and/or abused once marketed." In other words, nobody *knows* whether it's addictive, so psychiatrists are testing it on eleven million people to find out.

Unfortunately, we're already finding some evidence that Prozac causes a form of addiction—a form so subtle that both patients and psychiatrists have failed to recognize it for what it is. Psychiatrist Peter Kramer, after claiming that Prozac is a "relatively safe" drug that is not addictive ("patients do not crave Prozac, and there is no known withdrawal symptom"), states, in the same paragraph in his book *Listening to Prozac,* that "people who have experienced a good response to it are often leery about coming off medication, out of fear that they will return to their old way of feeling and behaving." A number of times in his book, Kramer describes attempting to take patients off of Prozac, only to find that they couldn't function without the drug: "the bottom had fallen out" of their lives, they were "not themselves" without Prozac. These patients' reactions, comments Charles Medawar, director of Social Audit (a British group that studies drug policies) hardly suggest that Prozac "is a drug that anyone can take or leave at will."

Medawar notes that Prozac is cleared from the body slowly, so that withdrawal symptoms may tend to peak well after the drug is stopped. Rather than recognizing these symptoms as effects of drug withdrawal, he comments in *Nature,* doctors and patients may misinterpret them as reemergence of disease—"and then see this as evidence of the effectiveness of the drug and of the need to continue treatment." Continued treatment, in turn, "would reinforce the dependence—and is exactly what happened with the benzodiazepines, barbiturates and all the rest."

Medawar's scenario is particularly alarming because most of the people taking Prozac *had no significant mental problems to begin with.* Many Prozac users are what psychiatrists refer to as "YAVISes"—*y*oung, *a*ttractive, *v*erbal, *i*ntelligent, and *s*uccessful people. YAVISes have always been the favorite patients of psychotherapists because there's nothing wrong with them that a little sympathetic talk can't help cure. But psychiatrists have been too willing to go along with these patients' belief that simply being normal isn't good enough, and too quick to hand out prescriptions for a drug whose potential for addiction isn't yet known.

DSM cooperates in this process by including categories such as "dysthymia" and "adjustment disorder," both of which can be stretched to fit just about anyone experiencing mild irritability, moodiness, or minor job or personal problems. Psychiatrists are increasingly expanding DSM's flexible categories to include milder and milder symptoms, and are pushing Prozac for normal personality variants such as shyness or overspending, which aren't symptoms of any "mental" problem at all. In effect, psychiatrists are defining normal behaviors as abnormal simply because medication alters them. Even Peter Kramer, Prozac's biggest proponent, worries about this phenomenon of "diagnostic bracket creep," saying that "we may mask the issue [of using drugs to create designer personalities] by defining less and less severe mood states as pathology, in effect saying, 'If it responds to an antidepressant, it's depression.'" In short, doctors are beginning to treat normal life problems with drugs—exactly what illegal drug users do. If you're fed up with life, bored with your job, or depressed over your own mortality, there's no longer any need to erase those bad feelings with marijuana or cocaine; you can do it legally now, with Prozac.

Prozac users themselves often seem uneasy with its use as an easy fix for life's woes. "A low-grade terminal anomie, a sense of alienation or disgust or detachment, the collective horror at a world that seems to have gone so very wrong, is not a job for antidepressants," says author Elizabeth Wurtzel (who, incidentally, takes Prozac for a DSM label of "depression," but is appalled at how many of her friends take the drug for what she calls "low-level sorrow"). "Just as our parents quieted us when we were noisy by putting us in front of the television set," she says in *Prozac Nation*, "maybe we're now learning to quiet our own adult noise with Prozac."

It's one thing when a physician prescribes a potentially addictive drug in an attempt to ease the symptoms of patients who have brain dysfunctions that *cannot currently be diagnosed or treated*. But it's another thing entirely to risk creating dependency in perfectly healthy individuals.

We don't know yet, of course, that Prozac users will become dependent on the drug. We also don't know that they won't. What we do know is that, in the past, whenever psychotropic drugs have been pronounced safe and nonaddictive, those making the pronouncements were unduly optimistic.

"The clear message of history," Medawar says, "is to beware of any explosive, mass demand for a psychoactive drug—and never to forget that patients don't crave so long as doctors readily prescribe."

It's easy to finger psychiatrists (and other doctors who misprescribe psychotropic drugs) as the villains in the overdrugging of normal Americans. But much of the responsibility lies with patients as well. As Richard Hughes and Robert Brewin note in *The Tranquilizing of America*, "the fault lies also with people who seek an easy way out, individuals who trust too much in a man [or woman] in a white coat and who do not ask pertinent questions." A patient who accepts a prescription for Prozac as a panacea for a less-than-perfect life is as irresponsible, in many ways, as a person who accepts drugs from a street-corner dealer. Remember: no one is holding you down and forcing Prozac down your throat.

Ritalin and Other "Kid Drugs"

The use of Prozac to treat patients with no discernible disorders worries me, but what concerns me even more is the drugging of a million or more children with methylphenidate (Ritalin). The morality of administering an amphetamine-like drug to such a massive number of undiagnosed or mislabeled children is questionable. So is the message we're sending them: that amphetamines and similar drugs are a solution to everything from serious medical problems to minor fidgeting.

It's puzzling that medical and educational systems, which invest so much effort in campaigning against illegal drug use, are in the forefront of this legal drug epidemic. The pro-Ritalin pressure brought to bear on parents of "hyperactive" children, both by schools and by doctors, is tremendous, and parents are giving in to it. Daniel Safer and John Krager reported, in 1988, that surveys of school nurses in one U.S. county revealed "a consistent doubling of the rate of medication treatment for hyperactive/inattentive students every four to seven years," and the same surveys indicated that the drug was frequently being prescribed not just for hyperactivity, but also for nonhyperactive learning-impaired students. Children are being placed on the drug at earlier and earlier ages; 200,000 prescriptions for Ritalin and other stimulants were written in 1993 for pre-school-age children, although the *Physician's Desk Reference* (PDR) specifically states that "Ritalin should not be used in children under six years, since safety and efficacy in this age group have not been established."

Yet there is little difference between the drug that doctors and school officials are pushing parents to accept and the drugs they're trying to keep out of the schoolyards. Ritalin's addictive nature has been common knowledge for decades; in 1971, the U.S. Department of Justice Bureau of Narcotics and Dangerous Drugs put Ritalin under hard narcotics controls because of its addictive nature. Sweden banned Ritalin altogether in the 1960s, because of widespread abuse by children and teens.

In the United States, Ritalin abuse appears to be on the rise. T. Parran and D. Jasinski recently reported on 22 Ritalin abusers, 9 of whom were parents of children taking the drug for hyperactivity. Hayley Carter and William Watson described 29 patients admitted to a single emergency room after abusing "Ts and Blues," a combination of Ritalin and the painkiller pentazocine, taken intravenously. In another report, Rodney Schmidt and colleagues described the growing incidence of emphysema in intravenous Ritalin abusers, apparently caused by talc from the pills. Even taken by itself, in pill form, Ritalin is popular; drug dealers can make a profit of more than $400 selling a 100-pill prescription of the drug on the streets.

Prescribing a drug with Ritalin's addictive potential to "learning disabled" or "hyperactive" children on the basis of vague DSM labels, rather than diagnosing and correcting the problems underlying their symptoms, is an extremely poor medical decision—especially because these children are already at extreme risk of developing serious substance abuse problems. (A recent study, by Patricia Hardman and Donald Morton, found that 98 percent of subjects randomly selected in a drug and alcohol rehabilitation center were labeled as having learning disabilities, and 89 percent were labeled as having attention deficit disorder.) The *Physician's Desk Reference* warns that Ritalin is dangerous for patients at risk of drug abuse because "such patients may increase dosage on their own initiative."

And what about psychiatrists who prescribe Ritalin for children who have *no* problems? As I've mentioned, it's far too easy, given the elastic criteria for "hyperactivity," to label perfectly normal children as hyperactive and drug them with Ritalin. The message we're sending these children is that even normal feelings—squirminess, frustration, boredom—are reasons to reach for drugs. Schools, doctors, and parents sometimes go a step further: they punish, scold, or intimidate children who attempt to get out of taking the drug. In effect, they're saying that it's bad *not* to take drugs.

Children taking Ritalin get the message that mind-altering drugs are beneficial rather than harmful; in addition, many of these children come to associate drug use with being liked, and being praised by parents and teachers for good behavior. With their drug use being reinforced at every turn, it's only natural that many of these children turn to other drugs when life gets difficult. "This abuse of drugs for 'medicinal' purposes in school children cannot help but predispose them to amphetamine, marijuana, heroin, and cocaine addiction later in life," says author and researcher Harris L. Coulter. "If over a million school children are taking Ritalin or an amphetamine every day from the teacher in the classroom, why should they not take something stronger from the stranger on the street?"

The same goes for teenagers whose psychiatrists prescribe antidepressants and other drugs for mild symptoms of maladjustment. Adolescents and young adults are particularly vulnerable to the seductive message that drugs can handle life problems, because they're at an age where even minor problems—from dating woes to acne—seem tragic and insurmountable. Giving antidepressants to these adolescents tells them that the painful process of growing and maturing is abnormal, and that this process can be easily circumvented by taking drugs.

But the hormonal fluctuations, neurotransmitter shifts, and body changes that occur in adolescence, although they tend to throw teens out of whack for a while, are natural and necessary biological steps in the transition from childhood to adulthood, and they shouldn't be artificially circumvented. More importantly, all adolescents have to work through the *emotional* issues of growing up. Saddling them with a chemical dependency, and putting them at greater risk of illegal drug abuse as well, isn't going to help.

If you want proof, just ask one teenager I know, who was put on drugs by a child psychiatrist for what I considered to be normal "growing pains." At the time he first saw the psychiatrist, this handsome, strapping 15-year-old was a terrific soccer player, got B's in school, and was suffering from nothing more than the mild angst of a normal teen making the transition from childhood to young adulthood. In short, he was about as normal as a teenager gets. But his parents, convinced by the psychiatrist that the boy's "dysthymia" (a DSM term for mild "depression") could be dangerous, agreed to treat him with imipramine, an antidepressant. Four years later, he's unable to stop taking the medication because he experiences severe withdrawal symptoms whenever he tries.

Would this young man have survived his mildly traumatic adolescence without this drug? Absolutely. Would he have been better off suffering a few emotional bruises, instead of having a chemical cushion? Again, absolutely. There's no avoiding the hard knocks of life. Try to avoid them by taking drugs, and you'll wind up paying—often a high price—later on.

The Self-Medicating Abuser

In addition to causing many cases of prescription drug addiction, psychiatrists generally have a poor track record in *treating* addiction to street drugs. Ironically, a common approach to treating an addict is to prescribe more drugs! Many psychiatrists fail to recognize that numerous cases of drug abuse, particularly in teens and young adults, are desperate attempts to self-medicate physical disorders that need to be diagnosed and treated.

One of my young patients, for instance, was smoking marijuana on a regular basis. An affable 17-year-old with a contagious grin and a quick wit, Eric fit the beach bum "druggie" stereotype:

blond hair in a ponytail, a surfer's tan, and typical "Valley" speech—"Like, when I surf, my knee hurts? And, like, the water makes it feel better? You know?" On evaluation, however, I found that Eric wasn't doing drugs just to fit in with the beach crowd. He was suffering from chronic, low-grade aches in his knees and other joints, which the marijuana eased considerably (as did the surfing, because water soothes sore joints). Further evaluation revealed that Eric was suffering from poststreptococcal arthritis, a common aftereffect of rheumatic fever. I prescribed penicillin, which successfully controlled acute flare-ups of his condition—certainly a more useful treatment than marijuana! (Conversely, the marijuana was probably far less harmful than the neuroleptic drugs a DSM-oriented doctor would have prescribed for him.)

Any time a teenager is abusing drugs or alcohol, a careful evaluation is called for. Although many cases of drug abuse stem from the pressures of adolescence, others are attempts to treat painful or unpleasant symptoms of physical disorders. Common (and frequently undetected) disorders that teens attempt to mask with drugs include mononucleosis, anemia, subclinical malnutrition, and lingering pain from injuries. None of these disorders will be diagnosed if a patient is simply labeled by a DSM-oriented psychiatrist as having a "psychoactive substance use disorder" and placed on yet more drugs.

Similarly, a DSM label of "alcohol use disorder" reveals nothing about *why* an individual became an alcoholic. Many people overuse alcohol in an attempt to self-medicate chronic pain—particularly the pain of back injuries or arthritis. And a significant percentage of alcoholics suffer from anxiety, panic disorders, agoraphobia, or other behavioral symptoms that indicate the presence of underlying physical disorders. (A recent study, for instance, found that 44 percent of hospitalized alcoholics suffered from symptoms of anxiety.) Treating the alcoholism, without attempting to diagnose the underlying dysfunction that caused the patient to drink, is generally fruitless.

The Stress Myth

Psychiatrists commonly cite "the stressful society we live in" as a reason for illegal drug use. And, ironically, one of the primary reasons psychiatrists prescribe potentially addictive psychoactive drugs is to help patients combat stress. In fact, Xanax—which, as I've discussed, is a dangerous and highly addictive drug—is being prescribed by many doctors as a "stress pill." But the entire concept of stress as a "disorder," now enshrined in DSM-IV, is seriously flawed.

In the first place, life has always been stressful. People who lived through plague epidemics in the Middle Ages, or famines in the 1800s, or two world wars in the 1900s, would find it hard to sympathize with the modern-day belief that "things weren't as stressful in the past." And people who say we're more rushed today than in the past are forgetting that, for hundreds of years, people literally worked from sunup to sundown just to keep body and soul together—and there was no "safety net" to catch them if they failed. Our lives may not be stress-free, but they are probably less stressful than those of our forebears.

In the second place, a reasonable amount of stress is *good* for you. In fact, lack of stress may be more harmful to physical and mental health than high stress levels: many busy executives thrive for years on a high-pressure schedule, only to drop dead weeks after beginning a relaxing retirement. Severe, chronic, long-term stress can indeed be harmful, but most of us don't even come close to reaching critical stress levels except on rare occasions. The popular impression that the majority of us are suffering terrible consequences from everyday stress—an impression reinforced by the large numbers of patients labeled by psychiatrists as having "stress disorders"—is simply not true.

"Each stage of life presents its special stresses," physician Eve Bargmann and colleagues note in *Stopping Valium*. "This is perfectly normal and consistent with our understanding of people as constantly growing, developing beings. . . . Stress as an abnormal condition to be treated with a pill has been, for the most part, a creation of the drug industry, which promotes sales by convincing doctors that patients coping with difficult life situations must take medication to dull their response to those circumstances."

This drug company myth—that everyday stress is a "sickness" requiring brain-altering drugs—has been pushed for decades in pharmaceutical ads, often with tremendous success. Some of the pharmaceutical industry's efforts to promote the concept of universal, debilitating stress have been almost laughable—for instance, this 1970 ad for Librium:

> The Sixties. It is ten years since Librium became available. Ten anxious years of aggravation and demonstration, Cuba and Vietnam, assassination and devaluation, Biafra and Czechoslovakia. Ten turbulent years in which the world-wide climate of anxiety and aggression has given Librium—with its specific calming action and its remarkable safety margin—a unique and still growing role in helping mankind meet the challenge of a changing world.

More recent promotions, while not so hyperbolic, still suggest that anxiety and stress, in and of themselves, are diseases and must be drugged away. And psychiatrists (and other doctors) are still falling for this message—as are their patients. They're making a big mistake that can have dangerous or even fatal consequences.

I recommend that we stop thinking of everyday stress as a frightening, debilitating process and recognize that it's a normal part of life. We should talk about the "challenges" of life, or the "exciting experiences" of life, rather than the "stress" of everyday events. And, for those people who can't handle a moderate amount of stress without turning to drugs or alcohol, I recommend a comprehensive medical and neurological examination. Their problem often is not the stress in their environment, but a physical disorder—anything from sleep apnea to an undiagnosed virus—that is sapping their strength and reducing their ability to deal with life and its challenges.

What I don't recommend, for anyone, is a DSM label of "stress disorder" and a prescription for dangerous and potentially addictive antianxiety drugs. If stress is intolerable, a doctor must ask why—and ask what else is going on with the patient.

Trauma and PTSD

I've been talking here about common, run-of-the-mill stress. But what about people who experience major traumas—fires, floods, tornadoes, bombings, earthquakes, and bridge collapses? We've been led to assume, by the psychiatric "crisis teams" sent almost immediately to any disaster scene, that people suffer severe psychic wounds from experiencing such traumas—or even from being in the general vicinity when they occur. DSM-IV categorizes the symptoms most survivors experience following a disaster as "acute stress disorder," suggesting that they are pathological and require treatment. But are these people really suffering from a "disorder" requiring psychotherapy and the use of potentially addictive medications? And are they really at great risk of suffering long-term consequences from their trauma? The answers, surprisingly, are "No," and "No."

Let's look at the DSM-IV description of acute stress disorder. According to the manual, this condition lasts a *maximum of four weeks* and causes numbing, detachment, a sense of "being in a daze," "derealization," "depersonalization," and an inability to recall events surrounding the traumatic experience. "Victims" have nightmares and/or flashbacks, become distressed in the presence of reminders of the trauma, tend to avoid situations or objects that arouse recollections of the trauma, are anxious, and have difficulty functioning at work or at home.

Admittedly, these symptoms aren't pleasant. But not every unpleasant thought or emotion we experience is a "disorder" that must immediately be treated with medication and psychotherapy. Some negative emotions (stress reactions among them) are hardwired into us biologically, and for very good reason: they enhance our survival. The anxiety and fear we experience following a trauma are, in effect, nature's way of telling us to take all possible measures to avoid similar traumas in the future. The sense of numbness and the depersonalization that often occur during or shortly after a trauma are most likely the body's way of allowing us to put our emotions on hold until it's safe to sort them out. These reactions may not be fun, but they're not pathological. In fact, we have names for people who can witness shocking events *without* experiencing strong psychological reactions: we call them "psychopaths," "sociopaths," and "perverts."

Although people normally have strong negative reactions immediately following a trauma, evidence suggests—contrary to the claims of "trauma specialists"—that these reactions usually do not lead to long-term mental distress. In fact, people seem to weather even severe crises pretty well. A long-term study of tornado survivors in Xenia, Ohio, for instance, found that:

> . . . there was an extremely low rate of severe mental illness, if any at all, as a consequences of the tornado. On the contrary . . . a large percentage of the people had extremely positive reactions to the disaster. Eighty-four percent of the people claimed that their experiences had shown them they could handle crises better than they thought; and 69% reported that they felt they had met a great challenge, and were better off for it . . . ." [cited by E. L. Quarantelli, in *Trauma and Its Wake*]

Researchers at several other disaster sites have noted similar long-term effects. In fact, some reported that the incidence of mental hospital admissions, crime, and marital discord tended to *drop* slightly after a natural disaster. This research raises questions as to whether the hordes of psychiatrists and psychologists who descend on flood- or earthquake-ravaged towns do good, or simply add to the residents' problems by labeling them as victims. And it raises more serious questions about the practice of prescribing drugs to normal individuals suffering from time-limited symptoms of anxiety following a disaster.

I also have questions about the new DSM "diagnosis" of posttraumatic stress disorder (PTSD), because a large number of people labeled with posttraumatic stress disorder suffer from brain dysfunctions blamed erroneously on past stressful experiences. Rachel, the concentration camp survivor I mentioned in Chapter 1, who was believed to be suffering from her war experiences but actually had typhus, is a good example.

So is another patient of mine, a police officer named Amanda, who underwent a bitter divorce and spent months of her time, and thousands of dollars, battling her ex-spouse for custody of her three children. Amanda eventually won her custody fight and settled into a normal routine of work and life as a single mom, but she continued to feel "not quite myself." "I was tired all the time," she said. "The kids would want to go to a movie or McDonald's, and all I'd want to do was sleep." She found herself snapping at her fellow officers over trivial incidents, and she realized she was becoming "a complete shrew" at home. She even began wondering whether her husband was right: Was she fit to be a mother? "Above all," she said, "I worried about my judgment on the job. When you're a cop, you have to be on top of things all the time or you could get someone killed."

Thinking she might have a "mental" problem, Amanda visited a psychiatrist, who labeled her as having depression and posttraumatic stress disorder resulting from the trauma of her divorce. "At first, I was relieved," she said, "because I didn't have to feel guilty about my behavior any more. The doctor told me PTSD happened to lots of people going through divorce." She underwent months of expensive psychotherapy, and took several powerful and potentially addictive drugs. But Amanda's initial relief and optimism faded as time went on. As she told me a year later, "I'm not getting any better—I'm getting worse."

And indeed, Amanda *was* getting worse—because her symptoms weren't caused by the divorce, stressful as it was. They were caused by diabetes mellitus, for which she needed insulin therapy.

I put Amanda on insulin, instructed her on following a proper diet, and started her on a good exercise program. She's doing fine now, and has regained her confidence in herself as a police officer and as a mom. But she wouldn't be fine if she had kept taking addictive drugs as a "treatment" for her diabetes.

It's important to note here that Amanda, like many "posttraumatic stress disorder" patients I've seen, had clear-cut, unmistakable symptoms of disease. She was thirsty, she itched, and she was losing weight in spite of a healthy appetite. In addition, she had a family history of diabetes, and all of her children had weighed over ten pounds at birth—one of the warning signs of diabetes. She had frequent vaginal infections, her cuts took longer than normal to heal, and an eye exam showed changes commonly associated with early diabetic stages. In short, Amanda was a textbook case of early-stage diabetes, yet her psychiatrist overlooked all of these symptoms simply because her "mental" problems could easily be blamed on a past trauma.

It's easy to "diagnose" posttraumatic stress disorders in such cases, because virtually everyone has experienced a major life trauma at one time or another. (And DSM conveniently includes a category called "delayed onset" PTSD, meaning that therapists can blame almost any trauma, no matter how distant, for a patient's symptoms.) Generally, however, such attributions are false. A trauma—particularly a trivial one, or one from the distant past—does not cause severe behavioral and emotional problems, unless an individual's brain functioning is already compromised. Even in cases where long-term psychiatric symptoms appear to stem from severe trauma—for instance, in Vietnam veterans—patients with the worst symptoms appear to have been those who had the most adjustment problems before the trauma occurred, again suggesting the presence of underlying biological risk factors. A large-scale study reported by Paula Schnurr and her colleagues, in the *American Journal of Psychiatry*, for instance, reveals that high precombat levels of introversion, paranoia, depression, and other behavioral problems—all likely indicative of underlying brain dysfunction—predicted either the development or the severity of symptoms experienced by those labeled as having PTSD.

In short, symptoms of PTSD frequently appear to be due less to the trauma itself than to a neurologically impaired individual's inability to deal with trauma and stress. Thus, medication and psychotherapy are ineffective treatments; the underlying neurological abnormality needs to be diagnosed and treated.

Most reactions to stressful events are normal and in fact beneficial, not pathological. When they do become abnormal, the culprit is often an underlying biological dysfunction rather than the stressful situation itself. Psychiatrists merely complicate such cases by assigning a DSM label and prescribing harmful and potentially addictive drugs—an all too common occurrence.

Misguided Compassion

If stress is normal and benzodiazepines are dangerous, and if benzodiazepines don't "treat" stress anyway, then why do psychiatrists and other doctors continue to prescribe these drugs for stress? Apparently, they feel obligated to "help" the stressed patient in some way, and benzodiazepines are the easiest method. It hurts any compassionate doctor to send a patient away "stressed out" or suffering, even if that stress or suffering is normal. And because drug companies have succeeded in minimizing the risks of benzodiazepines and other addictive prescription drugs, doctors may sincerely believe that they are doing their patients little or no harm. (Bear in mind that most of the information doctors receive about drugs comes from drug companies, which aren't afraid to distort or conceal negative findings.) Furthermore, doctors are often misled by "official" figures on benzodiazepine addiction, which are gross underestimates—largely because patients who have been maintained on the drugs for years aren't considered as "addicted." Doctors don't know their patients are addicts until those patients try to quit—something that won't happen as long as the prescriptions keep coming.

In the end, however, the responsibility for uncontrolled prescribing rests with the doctor in charge of the prescription pad. Patients can clamor for drugs all they want, and pharmaceutical companies can spend millions to promote them, but they still won't be used unless doctors write the prescriptions. Doctors who don't prescribe benzodiazepines and other addictive drugs rarely regret it; those who do prescribe them, and later learn the consequences, often do. Their remorse is summed up eloquently by British practitioner J. Stevens, writing in *Prescribers Journal:*

> In 20 years of practice, I am unaware of ever having helped a patient by prescribing a hypnotic [a benzodiazepine, barbiturate, or other "sleeping pill"], but I have written many such prescriptions and continue to do so. By prescribing hypnotics, I have caused much misery and harm and prevented many people, including myself, from taking a more positive attitude to a common symptom. I have no doubt caused dependency and habituation on a wide scale. . . . Experience has taught me, very slowly, much that my clinical teachers did not.

Millions of patients like Mrs. Li, and thousands of doctors like Dr. Stevens, have learned the hard way that benzodiazepines and similar drugs don't cure disease or solve life problems. If you're ever offered these drugs—or if you're a physician considering prescribing them—I hope you'll learn from their experiences, rather than repeat them.

CHAPTER 5

What's *Really* Wrong with You?

Why It's Not All in Your Head

If the brain does not constitute the basis of the mind, what does?

Michael Rutter,
in the *Journal of Child Psychology and Psychiatry*

The mind–body dichotomy which has plagued medicine for generations
is nonsense, as it opposes the body with the activity and function of
the brain, part of the body. This is like creating a dichotomy between
the whole of a car and the activity of its engine.

E. Fuller Torrey,
in *The Death of Psychiatry*

ONE OF THE SCARIEST BOOKS I'VE READ RECENTLY IS *I'M Not Crazy*, by a young woman named Frances Deitrick. Fran describes how she changed in a few short months from a happy-go-lucky "golden girl" into a raving, hallucinating "schizophrenic." She tells about her blinding headaches, her irrational behavior, her sudden hot and cold spells, and her despair when she could no longer make sense of voices, faces, or her own thoughts. She tells about how she nearly died, saved only by dangerous radiation treatments that eradicated the tumor growing on her brain.

But those aren't the scariest parts.

The *really* scary part of Fran's story is what happened to her when her tumor first started causing her brain to malfunction. Following a car accident, probably a result of her disoriented state, Fran was taken to a local hospital and then admitted to a psychiatric facility. There, she was told she had an "emotional" problem, and she was labeled as having schizophrenia and atypical bipolar disorder. Her constant pleas that she was suffering from "brain seizures"—her description for the bizarre sensations she experienced—fell on deaf ears. She apparently had no thorough medical workup, and her only treatment—other than regular doses of tranquilizers and Thorazine—consisted of group therapy designed to help her deal with her "mental" problem. Time and time again, Fran's doctors told her, literally, that her problem was "all in her head."

Finally, after months, Fran was rescued by an unlikely knight. A physician who was not assigned to her case pulled her aside one day and said, "I don't think you're crazy." He was right: the MRI he ordered confirmed that a rare tumor called a pontine glioma was responsible for her symptoms. Luckily, Fran was diagnosed before the tumor became incurable, and her treatment was successful. When she later confronted one of the doctors at the psychiatric hospital who had failed to diagnose her—and had subjected her to months of worthless group therapy—he replied that he knew how she felt, and suggested, "Why don't you come to my Group to get everything off your chest."

Unfortunately, such stories aren't rare. Thousands of patients like Frances Deitrick are receiving labels and psychotherapy when they need diagnosis and treatment.

The Limitations—and Dangers—of Psychotherapy

So far we've looked at the perils of psychotropic drugs, the favorite treatment method of DSM-oriented psychiatrists. But their second favorite method, psychotherapy—although it can benefit some patients—can be just as dangerous when it's misunderstood and misused. And unfortunately, that's a common occurrence. Thousands of people suffer or even die because psychotherapy is being used in place of, rather than as an adjunct to, medical diagnosis and treatment.

Prescribing psychotherapy for a patient whose symptoms stem from a serious biological problem, without diagnosing and treating the problem, is as foolish as prescribing psychotherapy for a patient having a heart attack. Although psychotherapy is very helpful in some circumstances (which I'll discuss later), it is *not a definitive medical treatment* for brain dysfunction. In fact, most psychotherapy these days isn't even provided by doctors, but by psychologists, social workers, and other nonmedical therapists.

It won't do a patient any good to develop insight into his or her problems, if they're actually caused by a biological abnormality that's going to keep getting worse. Yet modern psychiatrists, trained in the three-step DSM method—pick a label, prescribe a drug, refer for therapy—frequently substitute psychotherapy for medical treatment. In fact, drugs and psychotherapy are the *only* two treatments commonly prescribed by DSM-oriented psychiatrists. Read the *DSM-IV Casebook,* and you'll find that referrals for psychotherapy are an expected and approved treatment for patients in most DSM categories. Thus, if you're a psychiatric patient, you're almost bound to be referred, at some time or another, to a therapist.

There are, as I'll discuss later, times when a psychiatrist *should* refer a patient for psychotherapy or counseling. And there are times when psychotherapy can have an impact on brain dysfunction—although not for the reasons most of its practitioners believe. (More on that later as well.) I refer a number of patients to counselors and psychotherapists, often with very good results. But patients who are referred for such therapies should understand the limitations of both the therapies and the therapists.

The most important limitation is that *psychotherapy will not cure brain dysfunction.* There is no way to talk yourself out of brain symptoms caused by a physical disorder. As Frances Deitrick discovered the hard way, tumors don't respond to "talk therapy"; neither do infections, toxins, or genetic diseases. Furthermore, by offering an easy out for the psychiatrist, psychotherapy often stymies the search for the biological roots of a patient's problems. The step from DSM "diagnosis" to psychotherapy is all too simple.

David Healy, in *The Suspended Revolution,* offers a classic example: a middle-aged woman who took an overdose of pills in an unsuccessful attempt to commit suicide. The patient, who was
admitted to a psychiatric unit, was clearly very disturbed. She ate
poorly, slept poorly, could not concentrate, was consumed with
guilt, and had no energy. Interestingly, she complained of one
other symptom: a severe vaginal pain, which had started 20 years
earlier, after the birth of a child. The pain, which was so severe it
forced her to stop having intercourse with her husband, also occurred when she drove over bumpy roads, or even when she sat in
a chair. No obvious reason for the pain could be found by doctors.

The case, Healy notes, seemed "almost too Freudian to be
true." Although the woman's husband was a boor, she claimed
that she was unable to divorce him because her pain made it impossible for her to live independently. Most of the hospital staff
felt it was obvious that the woman's pain was "functional"—a defense against having sexual relations with her husband—and that
her depression and guilt stemmed from her unhealthy dependency
on her spouse. If she hadn't encountered Healy, she might have
been given a DSM label of "depression" or "conversion disorder"
(hysteria) and spent the rest of her years in psychotherapy.

But Healy points out a clue that was overlooked by most of the
woman's doctors: in addition to her vaginal pain, she suffered
from a sharp pain in her big toe. Noting that "the vagina and the
big toe share the same nerve root," Healy states that "only a real
pain in the vagina, especially one involving the nerves to the
vagina, would be likely to cause a pain in the big toe too." He
concluded that the woman suffered from a condition called
postepisiotomy pain syndrome—lingering pain resulting from a
surgery performed during childbirth to enlarge the opening of the
vagina and aid delivery of the baby. This condition is being reported with increasing frequency in the medical literature, but is
still virtually unknown to many psychiatric professionals (and to
DSM). Psychotherapy was the wrong choice as a frontline treatment for this patient—although it may have helped her, later on,
to deal with the emotional fallout from her biological condition.

In another case, reported by Frederick Goggans and colleagues, in *Medical Mimics of Psychiatric Disorders,* a 27-year-old executive was hospitalized after attempting to kill herself by overdosing on antidepressants prescribed by her psychiatrist. The woman's suicide attempt—her second—followed a year of psychotherapy that had failed to relieve her fatigue, cognitive problems, and despondency. She was distraught that her suicide attempt was unsuccessful, and told her doctors that she would probably try to kill herself again.

Luckily, this woman's new doctors, unlike her previous ones, searched for the causes of her behavior. After evaluating her carefully, they determined that she suffered from hypothyroidism, a common cause of listlessness, sadness, and hopelessness, and they gave her thyroid supplements. Since then, she has been free of psychiatric symptoms and has thrived both personally and professionally.

Not all individuals are as lucky as Goggans' patient. Although she nearly killed herself waiting for a diagnosis, she at least got one—which is more than millions of other patients can say. Among the mislabeled are thousands of individuals with Tourette's syndrome (TS), a genetic disorder that causes tics, such as eye rolling or shrugging, and behavioral problems including hyperactivity, excessive anger, and compulsions. "Therapists who are not familiar with the spectrum of disorders in TS often produce psychological explanations to explain the behaviors they are seeing or hearing about," researcher David E. Comings says in *Tourette Syndrome and Human Behavior.* "Tics may be labeled 'acting out behaviors,' or 'the result of psychological problems,' or due to 'stress in the home.' . . . Obsessive-compulsive behaviors may be labeled 'efforts to protect oneself from some inner conflict.' Sexual touching or compulsive masturbation are often assumed to be 'the result of sexual abuse in the home.' The anger, which is often such an integral part of TS, may be thought of as due to 'a reaction to parental conflicts or divorce,' to 'compensate for feelings of inadequacy,' or to a long list of 'unresolved conflicts.'" Comings says that many patients he sees have undergone years of completely ineffective treatment by psychoanalytically oriented therapists, only to respond readily to proper medical treatment.

These cases are excellent examples of why *no* patient should be referred for psychotherapy before receiving a careful deductive differential diagnosis. Often, a thorough evaluation will lead to a diagnosis and treatment that will eliminate the need for therapy. For other patients, the evaluation will clarify the types of therapy most likely to be successful.

In addition to misdiagnosing brain dysfunction, psychotherapists often mislabel other bodily disorders as "functional" problems—even when a patient shows no sign of abnormal thoughts or emotions. Researcher Robyn Dawes reports a case involving a middle-aged man who came to a hospital complaining that he was growing breasts. When the man told the intake doctor at the hospital that he was depressed over his mother's recent suicide—certainly a normal reaction—the patient was transferred to a hospital psychiatrist and then placed in a locked psychiatric ward. Dawes notes, in *House of Cards,* "The staff members on that ward, many of them psychoanalytically trained, were fascinated by the delusion of growing breasts following a mother's suicide." Psychotherapy appeared to be the obvious remedy for the man's imaginary bosom.

Fortunately for this patient, a friend of Dawes, after being asked to consult on the case, requested the results of the man's physical exam. When told that none had been performed, he recommended one. The exam and subsequent tests revealed that the man suffered from Klinefelter's syndrome, a result of having one Y and two X chromosomes. "He was indeed growing breasts," Dawes says, "a common result of the syndrome." By the time the man's condition was diagnosed, he had spent six weeks of involuntary imprisonment in the hospital's psychiatric ward.

Another case of misguided therapy for a clearly physical problem, reported by psychologist Paula Caplan in *They Say You're Crazy,* involved a woman who suffered from severe pain before each menstrual period. "She was repeatedly told that there was nothing physically wrong with her," Caplan says, and that the pain "must be emotionally caused." It wasn't. Years later, when the woman had surgery for an unrelated problem, her surgeon found a massive amount of scar tissue caused by earlier pelvic inflammatory disease. Because her infection went untreated for so long, it's unlikely that she will ever be able to have children.

Psychiatry's Brain–Mind Fallacy

Why do so many patients get sent to therapy instead of receiving medical diagnosis and treatment? Because psychiatry believes in the false premise of the "brain–mind dichotomy." Since the time of Freud, psychiatry has promoted the belief that some mental symptoms are caused by a malfunctioning brain, while others spring from nebulous "psychic trauma." Furthermore, psychiatrists have long proclaimed that they, as experts on the "mind," can easily determine which mental symptoms are caused by physical dysfunction, and which are all in the patient's mind. A patient with an obvious brain tumor, for instance, may be diagnosed as having an "organic" disease, while a patient with exactly the same symptoms—but no obvious tumor—may be diagnosed as suffering from a bad childhood. And if a tumor shows up later, the psychiatrist can still blame a bad childhood; witness the case of Charles Whitman, who climbed a tower at the University of Texas in 1966 and shot 13 people to death. Witman's autopsy revealed an almond-sized malignant brain tumor that almost assuredly caused profound behavioral disturbance. Yet a psychiatrist and self-proclaimed "expert" on the case, when asked to comment, said that the tumor would not have affected Whitman's behavior, which he believed stemmed from personal problems.

The strange concept that a symptom such as sadness, hopelessness, or anxiety can stem either from a brain disorder or from a disembodied "mind" is a natural outgrowth of psychiatry's tortuous past. As I've noted, psychiatry—originally a biologically oriented medical field—was hijacked in the mid-1900s by Freudian and post-Freudian psychoanalysts who believed that psychiatric symptoms were caused by early childhood trauma, and that the brain played little or no role in "mental" disorders. Modern psychiatry claims to have dethroned the psychoanalysts in favor of biological approaches to treating mental illness, but this revolution is incomplete. The result, at least for now, is a mishmash of biological and psychological explanations for most psychiatric disorders—and a strange situation in which psychiatrists attempt to treat the brain with drugs, and the "mind" with therapy.

DSM, a manual written by a committee attempting to placate both biologically oriented psychiatrists and psychoanalysts (still a powerful force, despite their dwindling numbers), willingly buys into the concept of the brain–mind dichotomy. It accomplishes this, in a somewhat cowardly fashion, by refusing to take sides regarding the causes of many behavioral disorders. In fact, despite being labeled as a diagnostic manual, DSM does its best to avoid diagnosis altogether. Labels such as "narcissistic personality disorder" and "dissociative identity disorder" offer few hints as to the *causes* of patients' symptoms. Does the narcissistic patient have a brain tumor, or is she seeking the love her father denied her? Is the dissociative patient suffering from lead poisoning, or is he upset because his mother remarried? DSM-IV devotes only a few sketchy comments to causation in each section, leaving it up to individual psychiatrists to determine whether most patients are experiencing biological problems or psychic trauma.

DSM's brain–mind cop-out is embodied in its system of "diagnosis," in which patients are described on five different axes. These are:

Axis 1: A clinical disorder included in the DSM. (This is generally written in DSM "code," which looks something like this: "308.3: Acute Stress Disorder.")

Axis 2: Personality disorder or mental retardation.

Axis 3: General medical condition. (Note: Physical exams are usually skipped, or delegated to other doctors.)

Axis 4: Psychosocial and environmental problems.
Axis 5: Global assessment of functioning. (How well is the patient able to cope with work, family, home, and so on?)

The object of this system is to allow psychiatrists to say that they have considered all aspects of a patient's problem: biological, social, and psychodynamic. Let's see how this system works in real life. Take an imaginary 45-year-old female patient who has suddenly developed symptoms that include lethargy, irritability, and sadness. Her five-axis DSM "diagnosis" might look like this:

Axis 1: Phase of life problem.
Axis 2: Dependent personality.
Axis 3: Postmenopausal, obesity.
Axis 4: Severe. Recent divorce; lives alone.
Axis 5: (60) Moderate difficulty in social and occupational functioning.

What does this lengthy "diagnosis" tell us about our patient? Not much. We don't know if her recent emotional problems stem from hormonal imbalances linked to menopause. We don't know if both her obesity and lethargy are caused by metabolic problems. We don't know whether her "phase of life" problem is a normal and time-limited reaction to her divorce, or the result of brain dysfunction. In short, we don't know anything about the cause of her symptoms, and we certainly don't know how to treat them. This leaves her psychiatrist free to blame any cause—divorce, menopause, "life circumstance"—for her problems, and to prescribe either biological or psychotherapeutic intervention—or both.

Furthermore, each DSM category lists a handful of possible brain disorders to "rule out"—strongly implying that if these few conditions aren't present, whatever is left over may be "functional." (The category of "generalized anxiety disorder," for instance, lists only three or four specific biological disorders to rule out, even though the condition has dozens of well-known and well-documented physical causes.) Presumably, a psychiatrist who has ruled out the few biological conditions listed as possibilities under each DSM label is then free to decide whether a patient's problem involves the body or the "mind."

The result of such silliness is exactly what you'd expect: a complete lack of standards for treatment of brain dysfunction. A good example of this appeared recently in an article in *Psychology Today,* which simultaneously applauded two groups of psychiatrists treating patients suffering from panic attacks. One group is investigating the idea that panic attacks are caused by a respiratory "warning system" that is overly sensitive to oxygen deprivation. The other, a Freudian-oriented group of psychiatrists, insists that although patients may have some physiological abnormality, their real problem is "suffocating" parents who create children resentful of their parents but overly dependent on them. When these children grow up, the psychiatrists say, an authority figure or "powerful other" can trigger angry responses that frighten the patient into an anxiety attack.

Both of these groups may be wrong, but only one of them could possibly be right. Any other medical field would bet on the group with the most scientific evidence to support it. But DSM takes no stand as to the cause of panic disorder—and because DSM is the official "diagnostic" manual of the American Psychiatric Association, that means that psychiatry takes no stand on whether panic disorder is caused by physiological abnormalities or suffocating parents. In fact, DSM is noncommittal about both the causes and the treatments of virtually all "mental" disorders. (It's little wonder that there are still therapists—some on government payrolls—practicing exorcisms.)

Believe it or not, when DSM-III eliminated most references to causes of psychiatric disorders, it was considered a major step *forward* rather than a momentous step backward. But regressing from diagnosis to description is not progress. Correct diagnostic measures result in an ever-increasing understanding of disease causes, while labeling without regard to causation results in an ever more shallow system of identification and an ever less scientific system of treatment.

Functional Follies

In the introduction to DSM-IV, the authors claim to have ended the distinction between "organic" disorders (those known to be caused by brain dysfunction) and "functional" disorders (those with no known physiological cause, and therefore considered "all in the mind"). The distinction between organic and functional, they say, "implies a distinction between 'mental' disorders and 'physical' disorders that is a reductionistic anachronism of mind/body dualism." Hear, hear! Unfortunately, after saying this, DSM's authors go on to list a slew of labels that can only be considered functional. Here are some examples.

CONVERSION DISORDER

This DSM term (an updated term for "hysteria") is applied to patients who have symptoms suggesting neurological disorders or other medical problems, but who are treated as psychologically disordered because "the initiation or exacerbation of the symptom or deficit is preceded by conflicts or other stressors," and "the symptom or deficit cannot, after appropriate investigation, be explained by a general medical condition."

Unfortunately, the term is commonly used to write off the symptoms of patients (usually women) suffering from real and potentially dangerous physical diseases. Physicians Barry Fogel and Andrew Slaby have described the case of a woman who overdosed on opiates and went into a coma, but was misdiagnosed as "hysterical" in spite of her abnormal EEG and cerebral swelling.

Other frequent victims of DSM's "conversion disorder" label are women in the early stages of multiple sclerosis or lupus, which can initially present with vague physical complaints and/or behavioral symptoms. Even cancer can be labeled as a "mental" complaint: Patty Delaney Klafehn says it took her five years to get a diagnosis of Hodgkin's disease (a form of cancer that often is quite treatable if diagnosed early), largely because doctors believed her symptoms were psychosomatic. "I itched all over my body, had incredible pain in my arms and legs and felt tired all the time," she told *Redbook* writer Rita Baron-Faust. "But not one of those doctors ever did tests to see if I had Hodgkin's—even though, I found out later, severe itching is a common symptom of the disease." By the time her disease was diagnosed, it was in an advanced stage.

Then there was the case, reported by physician Joseph Wassersug, in *American Medical News,* of the woman with a tickle in her throat. When the woman told doctors she'd had the problem since childhood, when she'd swallowed a coin, they diagnosed her as "hysterical." One doctor told her, "It's your womb that's stuck in your throat, not a coin." But Wassersug was intrigued by her story. He put her in front of his office X-ray machine, and got a perfect picture of the coin that had been lodged in her throat tissue for more than sixty years!

CONDUCT DISORDER AND OPPOSITIONAL DEFIANT DISORDER

These DSM labels are often applied to children and teens who commit crimes, vandalize property, and/or "act out" against their parents or school authorities. The words used in these labels— *conduct, oppositional, defiant*—strongly suggest behavioral reactions to environmental influences, and psychiatrists frequently ascribe such problems to abusive or overly authoritarian parents. In most cases, however, there is a far more logical biological explanation.

In *Mind or Body,* physician Robert Taylor describes a patient whose teenage delinquency (including theft and assault) almost certainly would have earned him the label of "conduct disorder" from a DSM-oriented psychiatrist. The patient grew into a vindictive and demanding adult who abused his wife and children. After a particularly brutal assault on his wife, he was labeled as having "psychopathic personality" and committed to a criminal asylum. But the man didn't have "conduct disorder" or "psychopathic personality"; what he actually had was Huntington's chorea, a progressive neurological disorder that affected his muscle movements, speech, and brain. He died at age 32 from complications of this hereditary disorder—which wasn't diagnosed until a few years before his death, despite the fact that his mother had died of Huntington's chorea, and despite his own physical symptoms (which included difficulty walking, jerky arm movements, and facial grimaces).

Another disorder commonly mislabeled as conduct disorder is Tourette's syndrome (TS), a genetic disorder. Interestingly, TS is listed as a DSM-IV diagnosis; but conduct disorder is not listed as a symptom of TS, and TS is not mentioned as a cause of conduct disorder! Thus, a child without blatant signs of TS is likely to receive a label of conduct disorder instead. Researcher David Comings describes one such child:

> He had a lifelong history of severe behavioral problems. Multiple mental health workers had characterized him as argumentative, prone to violent temper tantrums, aggressive outbursts, physically and verbally abusive. . . . In spells of rage he has poked holes in walls and knocked the door off its hinges.

This boy, finally diagnosed by Comings, had been labeled as having childhood schizophrenia and "undersocialized, aggressive conduct disorder" by doctors who had overlooked his TS symptoms.

Conduct disorder is also a common misdiagnosis for children suffering from nutritional deficiencies. Physician Jun-Bi Tu and colleagues recently reported on two such children in the *Canadian Journal of Psychiatry*. Both children were labeled as conduct-disordered and treated with Ritalin or antidepressants. One had a history of "frequent aggressive outbursts, destructiveness, truancy, drug abuse, sexual acting-out, running away from home, [and] lying and stealing with no regard for other people." The other "had been charged with assault for violent outbursts and for threatening people with a knife . . . [and] was also considered to be a sexual offender against younger children." The second patient also suffered from hallucinations, had tried to choke his younger brother, and had threatened to commit suicide. A comprehensive evaluation by Jun-Bi Tu uncovered "striking iron deficiency" in both children, and treatment with iron supplements led to dramatic behavioral improvement.

Many other children labeled with "conduct disorder" actually have fetal alcohol syndrome (FAS), the leading nongenetic cause of mental retardation, and a major cause of learning disabilities and problem behavior. FAS, caused by alcohol exposure while the fetus is in the womb, is a very common disorder—yet it rates only a few dozen words in the DSM and is *not listed as a diagnostic category itself.* Children with severe cases of FAS have distinctive facial abnormalities and retardation, but those with milder cases generally go undiagnosed. Children with mild FAS suffer primarily from learning problems, attention problems, and impulsivity, but quite a few also exhibit significant behavioral problems such as bullying, sullenness, lying, cheating, or stealing. (A recent study by Ann Streissguth and her colleagues found that 62 percent of adolescents and adults with FAS exhibited significant behavior problems.) Of the more than 7,000 FAS children born every year, many are later adopted. Their adoptive families—frequently unaware that the children suffer from brain dysfunction—are often told that the children's "conduct disorder" or "oppositional defiant disorder" stems from the trauma of being adopted or from some failing on the part of the new family.

This is not surprising, because DSM-IV doesn't list FAS as a possible cause of conduct disorder. Nor does it list lead poisoning, Huntington's chorea, or dozens of other brain dysfunctions that can cause aggression and other behavior problems. Instead, it says:

> The following factors may predispose the individual to the development of conduct disorder: parental rejection and neglect, difficult infant temperament, inconsistent child-rearing practices with harsh discipline, physical or sexual abuse, lack of supervision, early institutional living, frequent changes of caregivers, large family size, association with a delinquent peer group, and certain kinds of familial psychopathology.

And oppositional defiant disorder, a label for similar but milder behaviors, is blamed primarily on "families in which child care is disrupted by a succession of different caregivers or . . . families in which harsh, inconsistent, or neglectful child-rearing practices are common."

So much for the "biological revolution" in psychiatry!

HYPOCHONDRIASIS

This label is applied to thousands of patients believed to be "making up" their symptoms. According to DSM, the label should be given to patients who continue to believe that they have serious illnesses, despite reassurances from doctors, negative examinations and test results, and apparent lack of disease.

But generally these patients have indeed developed a disease; their physicians simply haven't found it yet. One problem commonly labeled as hypochondria is peripheral neuropathy, a nerve condition that can cause numbness, tingling, hallucinations, and other symptoms easily dismissed as "mental." Another is Lyme disease, a tick-borne bacterial disease. In *Lyme Disease: The Great Imitator,* Alvin Silverstein and colleagues, who are specialists on the disorder, write about one typical patient who spent $20,000 in medical bills over three years before she found a doctor who believed that her symptoms were real. (This story brings up an interesting point. Lyme disease was only "discovered" in the late 1970s. It's logical to assume that there are dozens or even hundreds of similar disorders that medical science hasn't yet identified. How many such disorders are currently being labeled as "hypochondria"?) It's true that some patients, in a phenomenon known as *somatic compliance,* will embroider or elaborate on their symptoms. However, that's a natural reaction when one suffers from a vague, hard-to-define unwellness that is constantly dismissed by doctors as "nothing."

Neurologist Bruce Dobkin, in *Brain Matters,* describes a classic example of both "hypochondria" and somatic compliance. One of his patients, Carol, recited a laundry list of symptoms ranging from headaches and arm pains to blurred vision, weakness, dizziness, dry skin, and constipation. None of her symptoms could be verified through careful neurological evaluation, and Dobkin was about to give up and label Carol as a hypochondriac when, in the midst of her litany, she mentioned that "once when we were visiting friends, I guess I took off my pants in their living room, sat on the floor, and stuffed them under a sofa." Dobkin, curious, asked Carol if she'd been aware of doing this. She hadn't—and she related a string of similar incidents involving "dreamy" states and peculiar behavior such as urinating on herself, staring, and incomprehensible mumbling.

"Now the woman made some sense to me," Dobkin says. "She was not . . . a malingerer or a hypochondriac on a kamikaze mission against doctors. She clutched onto symptoms such as pain and dizziness because no one recognized her real symptoms as a disease." Further evaluation revealed, as he suspected, that Carol suffered from psychomotor seizures (which he documented with an EEG). For years they had gone undetected by her physicians, who had medicated her with Valium and antidepressants and referred her to therapy for her "hypochondria."

It's true that some patients' descriptions of symptoms are too bizarre to have a basis in fact. But even if no physical disorder exists and a patient still insists there is pain, then the patient can be said to be hallucinating—which in itself is a sign of a dysfunctional brain and should be investigated.

FACTITIOUS DISORDER

This DSM label states its bias up front rather than beating around the bush: the word "factitious" means "manufactured" or "artificial." Thus, the patient labeled as having a "factitious disorder" is actually labeled as a liar—or, in the words of DSM-IV, as someone who "intentionally produces or feigns [symptoms]" in an attempt to "assume the sick role." But although the symptoms of a patient with "factitious disorder" may be medically impossible, the patient is generally suffering from a diagnosable disorder. The key semantic error DSM-IV makes in describing such patients is in saying that they are *intentionally* feigning an illness—a statement no more true than saying a patient is intentionally having a hallucination. The behavior of an individual with "factitious disorder," like the behavior of a hallucinating patient, is clearly symptomatic of disturbed thought processes emanating from a dysfunctional brain.

A good example of misapplication of a "factitious" label involves a 35-year-old patient recently described by Gilles Fenelon and colleagues in the *British Medical Journal*. The patient's label was "Munchausen's syndrome," a variation of factitious disorder in which an individual continually visits hospitals seeking treatment of an acute illness that doesn't exist, and offering false medical histories to doctors. In this case, the man claimed to have had cataracts, a detached retina, glaucoma, alcoholism, cardiac arrhythmia, urinary infections, epilepsy, and diabetes. He was once caught rubbing a thermometer to raise the mercury to an abnormal reading. Most psychiatrists would believe DSM's explanation that the patient most likely had "a grudge against the medical profession," or "an important relationship with a physician in the past," and was in need of psychotherapy to work through emotional issues.

But a magnetic resonance image (MRI) scan ordered by Fenelon's group showed a more logical reason for the man's behavior. The scan revealed changes in the white matter of his brain that could be caused by multiple sclerosis, infections, toxic exposure, or vascular disorders. It's unlikely that treatment focusing on this patient's possible "grudges against the medical profession" would have changed his behavior, which almost certainly was caused by his abnormal brain.

I'm not naive enough to believe that all patients are entirely truthful about their symptoms. Like all doctors, I've examined patients suffering from "lawyer-itis"—a syndrome that occurs when a patient with a minor, accident-related symptom meets up with an eager attorney who senses an opportunity for a big payoff. For every schemer, however, there are dozens of patients with real, serious symptoms that have been dismissed as "factitious" (or as "malingering" or "hypochondria") by the psychiatric profession.

SOMATIZATION DISORDER

This label is applied to thousands of people suffering symptoms as diverse as irregular, heavy menstrual bleeding; heart palpitations; and chronic nausea, vomiting, and diarrhea. The term, most often applied to patients experiencing multiple symptoms in different body systems, is usually selected after an incomplete diagnostic workup shows no clear-cut medical problems. The authors of the *New Harvard Guide to Psychiatry* write that patients labeled as having somatization disorder are "highly dramatic and emotional in their description of their symptoms and suffering and are preoccupied with themselves, their bodies, and their illnesses," and that they "are usually resistant to the idea that their symptoms are the manifestation of emotional problems, and . . . are consequently refractory [resistant] to treatment involving the techniques of insight psychotherapy." This is not surprising. I would be emotional and resistant, too, if my doctor told me that my chest pains and chronic diarrhea were imaginary, and that I was being—to quote the *Guide*—"highly emotional, demanding, dramatic and manipulative" for disagreeing. A patient receiving a label of "somatization disorder" should find another physician who will perform a thorough workup for cancer, endometriosis, autoimmune disorders, and a multitude of other brain-affecting diseases that masquerade as "mental" illness.

"Functional": The Dysfunctional Diagnosis

Imagine the chaos if other physicians operated in the same manner as DSM-oriented physicians. Suppose, for instance, that the *Washington University Manual of Medical Therapeutics*—a standby of general practitioners—listed Valley fever and measles and melanoma, but refused to speculate as to the causes of these diseases, or to recommend methods of treatment. Or suppose that any disorder a cardiologist or gynecologist couldn't diagnose in an hour or so was considered to be "functional." Suppose, further, that patients who disagreed, insisting that they had real physical illnesses, were labeled as "demanding" and "manipulative" for seeking effective diagnoses and treatment.

(Actually, nonpsychiatric medicine does occasionally succumb to a belief in a "body–mind dichotomy." Asthma, peptic ulcers, and mitral valve prolapse—a heart condition that can cause symptoms of anxiety—were all, at one time or another, blamed on psychogenic factors. And cystitis, a bladder infection that causes excruciating pain and itching, was once blamed on female emotional instability! But, in general, nonpsychiatrists look longer and harder for a diagnosis before writing patients off as "mental cases.")

Although functional diagnoses are still quite popular with psychiatrists, they are in fact nondiagnoses. The idea that mental disorders can be divided into "organic" and "functional" categories ignores a fundamental fact: *the brain is the organ of behavior.* Libido, anger, joy, sadness, memory, speech, and all other human emotions and behaviors are subject to injuries, illnesses, or imbalances affecting brain cells (neurons). Any disruption of thought, emotion, or behavior *must begin in the brain.*

I'm not saying that behavior and emotion are not influenced by outside occurrences. If someone you love dies, you grieve. If you experience a happy event, you feel good. If you live in a violent neighborhood, you'll probably be more anxious than if you live in a peaceful area. *But your reactions to these events are constrained by the functioning of your neurons.* A normal brain will create normal sensations of anger, happiness, fear, or love; an abnormal brain will create wildly inappropriate reactions to the same situations. One can make an analogy to the heart muscle: a normal heart, while it may beat very quickly when a person is frightened and slowly during relaxing times, functions within normal limits. A person who dies of a heart attack after a minor scare was killed not by the event, but by his faulty heart.

Likewise, a college student who strips off all of her clothes and runs in front of a bus after flunking a test, or a teenager who responds to the death of his hamster by shooting up his house, cannot be said to be suffering from a "functional" disorder. In such cases, *an abnormal brain is producing abnormal reactions to situations a normal brain would react to much differently.* The bottom line: something is wrong with the brain.

It offends many people to suggest that our feelings and behaviors are products of our neurons rather than of an invisible mind, but the conclusion is unavoidable. Take away the brain, and you have no "mind." Alter the neurons in the brain, and the thoughts, behaviors, and emotions we attribute to the "mind" become distorted or nonexistent. Correct brain dysfunction, and thoughts, behaviors, and emotions become normal. Ergo, thoughts, behaviors, and emotions begin in the brain—or, more correctly, the billions of neurons that conduct messages in the brain. It is impossible to have a "mental illness" without a dysfunctional brain—and it is impossible to evaluate the "mind" without evaluating the brain. Furthermore, although there is an "unconscious," it originates—as does conscious thinking—from the neuron. Otherwise, the unconscious wouldn't exist.

"A mental 'disease' is said to be a 'disease' of the mind," psychiatrist E. Fuller Torrey notes in *The Death of Psychiatry.* "But a 'mind' is not a thing and so technically it cannot have a disease. 'Mind' is shorthand for the activity and function of the brain."

This doesn't mean that humans should think of themselves as mere machines—a depressing point of view. It means that we should acknowledge that our brains, honed over millions of years of evolution, are amazing tools that give us the ability to perform wonderful feats, from writing novels, to curing disease, to falling in love. "To say that our behavior is based on a vast, interacting assembly of neurons," Sir Francis Crick, the Nobel-prize-winning codiscoverer of DNA, says in *The Astonishing Hypothesis,* "should not diminish our view of ourselves but enlarge it tremendously."

Crick notes that philosophers have made little progress in understanding consciousness—what psychiatrists call "the mind" or "the psyche"—because "they are looking at the system from outside. . . . It is essential to think in terms of neurons, both their internal components and the intricate and unexpected ways they interact together. Eventually, when we truly understand how the brain works, we may be able to give approximate high-level accounts of our perceptions, our thinking, and our behavior."

The Uses of Psychotherapy

Because "mental" disorders are actually medical disorders, psychotherapy's role in treating them is limited. Therapy can't cure "mental" illness. It can't do anything to correct aberrant thinking stemming from a malfunctioning brain (although it can, as I'll discuss later, have a temporary effect on brain chemistry). There are, however, several things psychotherapy *can* do, sometimes very effectively.

THE THERAPEUTIC LISTENER

If anyone ever needed a sympathetic and understanding listener, it's a patient with a brain dysfunction. In addition to the burdens any major illness creates—financial pressures, family tensions, fears of disability or death—people with behavioral disorders face stigmatization by a society that describes people with brain dysfunction as "crazy," "nut cases," or "psychos." Friends and family aren't likely to accept schizophrenia or manic depression in the same casual way they accept a back injury or heart condition; in general, psychiatric conditions are hushed up as something shameful or embarrassing. As psychiatrist Abraham Twerski notes, in *Who Says You're Neurotic?*, "While people with asthma or arthritis bewail their condition (why me?), they generally do not go about feeling guilty about their misery. On the other hand, depressives not only suffer intensely but also feel profound guilt for being depressed, as if they were depressed by choice. Very often depressives will say, 'Why am I doing this to myself?'"

Furthermore, the person suffering from brain dysfunction isn't always easy to talk to; the wildly illogical talk, manic ramblings, or repetitiveness typical of patients with brain dysfunction can rapidly turn off even the most sympathetic listener. Thus, a person with a brain dysfunction often finds it difficult or impossible to talk openly with others about his or her problems.

A therapist can serve as an understanding, nonjudgmental listener, allowing the patient to vent negative feelings and achieve a catharsis. By affirming that a patient's brain dysfunction does not make the patient "bad" or "weak," a therapist can also help the patient regain dignity and self-respect. And, by suggesting practical and helpful ways for dealing with the problems a mental dysfunction creates, therapy can help a patient regain a sense of control over his or her life. Note that the therapist is dealing with the *normal emotional consequences* of a traumatic life event—sadness, fear, anxiety, anger—and not the abnormal output of the brain, which can't be altered by "talk therapy." As psychiatrist Jerrold Maxmen notes, "No one expects . . . psychotherapy to cure diabetes, yet it clearly helps patients deal with their diabetes. The same applies for helping patients deal with mental illness."

Therapy is a nonmedical treatment that doesn't address the patient's underlying brain dysfunction. Interestingly, however, therapy can help to relieve the very normal stress, anger, and fear a patient naturally experiences. In this very limited sense, therapy can alter brain chemistry.

Skeptical? Then do this quick exercise in the power of negative thinking. It requires only your imagination, for less than a minute. Imagine that you're driving in heavy, fast traffic and you see a large tarantula climbing onto your steering wheel and then crawling slowly up your bare arm. Concentrate intensely for a moment on this scary image, and pretend it's really happening. Now, imagine that you're home alone, you hear glass breaking, and then you see a burglar with a gun climbing through your window. In a moment, you and the burglar will be face-to-face.

If you really worked at this exercise, you changed your body chemistry and functioning. Your heart rate increased, your breathing changed, and you probably felt your skin crawl. All of these responses were caused by shifts in brain neurotransmitters—and they in turn caused further changes in the brain's chemical balance.

In a similar fashion, the bodily functions of a person with brain dysfunction are altered not only by the disorder, but also by the brain's normal reactions to it. An individual with a brain dysfunction quite naturally experiences abject terror at the idea of "going crazy." He or she also experiences anger, guilt, sadness, anxiety, and feelings of helplessness and hopelessness. All of these normal reactions, in turn, alter the chemistry of the body and the brain. Chronic anxiety, for instance, tends to make individuals breathe shallowly, which alters carbon dioxide levels; this change, in turn, alters the pH balance in the body, which can lead to sensations of panic. Chronic feelings of defeat and hopelessness alter levels of steroids, neurotransmitters, and other chemicals, causing distortions in thought and feeling. Anger alters levels of both neurotransmitters and hormones. Therapy, by relieving these normal but often counterproductive emotions, can also ameliorate their biochemical effects.

This is, by the way, a good reason why patients should be cautious about therapies that seek to blame poor parenting, early childhood trauma, or repressed memories for brain dysfunction. In addition to being wrong about the causes of "mental" disorders (see Chapter 6), therapies that dwell on past negative events are likely to exacerbate, rather than relieve, anxiety, anger, and other negative emotions—which, in turn, can exacerbate biochemical imbalances in the brain.

DEALING WITH "PROBLEMS IN LIVING"

Some people who visit psychiatrists have nothing wrong with their brains at all. Such patients may complain of unsatisfying jobs, difficulty getting along with their children, unfulfilling marriages, the grief of losing a loved one, or the difficulty of caring for a disabled family member. Their distress, while very real, has nothing to do with abnormal brain function; in fact, these patients' brains are responding quite correctly to less-than-satisfactory situations. In psychiatrists' terms, these patients have "issues" rather than "symptoms."

What these individuals often need, quite simply, is an unbiased and supportive listener. Many people get that kind of support from understanding friends, family members, or the local priest or bartender. But many others aren't lucky enough to have a stable network of supportive friends and family. Some people are dealing with special problems and situations that are difficult for others to understand—for instance, a spouse with Alzheimer's, or a child with Down syndrome. Still others need a little extra help in making decisions, or in breaking bad habits such as smoking or overeating.

For such people, therapy can be of great help. Grieving patients, for instance, often benefit enormously from sessions with therapists who allow them, quite simply, to feel *angry* at the person who has died. This process can help patients recover not only from the initial sadness and hopelessness that naturally follow a terrible loss, but also from "anniversary" reactions—annual recurrences of sadness on the date a loved one died.

Although therapy can be helpful, don't pay good money to a psychiatrist for it. A few forms of therapy, such as behavior modification for severely retarded or autistic individuals, may require a highly trained therapist. For most forms of therapy, however, nurses, social workers, and clergy are every bit as effective as psychiatrists and psychologists. A review of 24 studies by D. M. Stein and M. J. Lambert, in *Clinical Psychology Review,* for instance, found no evidence that trained, experienced therapists had any more success in helping people than inexperienced therapists did.

And H. H. Strupp, who assigned disturbed college students either to highly trained analysts or to college professors who had no training at all but had warm personalities, found that there was no difference in outcome between the two groups of students.

Some research, in fact, suggests that self-administered therapy, using techniques learned from books or tapes, can be as effective as treatment by a trained therapist. F. Scogin and colleagues, in 1990, examined 40 studies that compared self-help programs to therapist-administered treatments for habit control, depression and anxiety, phobias, parenting difficulties, and sex, sleep, and memory problems. The differences in outcome between subjects using self-help techniques and subjects using trained therapists, they reported in *Psychological Science,* were not significant.

Studies also show that support groups can be as effective as therapy, both for people with "problems of life" and for people with actual brain dysfunction. (Alcoholics Anonymous, for instance, has as good a track record as professional therapies for substance abuse.) In addition, support groups can be an excellent source of information about treatments and resources. You don't even have to leave your home to join such a group, thanks to the many computer support groups springing up around the country (and the world). A significant advantage of these high-tech groups is that they allow people with rare problems to meet each other; for instance, one computer network was established by high-functioning individuals with autism.

Whether you choose a professional therapist or take the self-help route, it's important to avoid therapies focusing on blame and recrimination. Negative therapies, as we'll see in the next chapter, can turn even minor problems into major life crises for you and your family. If you were abused as a child, or raped, or otherwise seriously traumatized, talking about the experience can help. But if you haven't experienced any out-of-the-ordinary life traumas, there's little evidence that wallowing in self-pity over long-ago slights will do you any good.

One more caution: if you see a therapist to discuss problems in living, and there is nothing wrong with you, don't let your therapist "pathologize" your problems. This happens more often than you'd think, because mental health professionals are trained to focus on aberration, not on normality. (As the old psychoanalysts' joke goes, "The person who arrives at a party early is anxious; the one who arrives on time is compulsive; and the one who arrives late is hostile.") Studies show that plenty of perfectly normal people walk away from their therapists with labels suggesting that they are in serious trouble. And, as I've noted, DSM's ever-increasing list of conditions makes it easy for therapists to spot pathology where none exists. Consider the following DSM "diagnoses:"

- *Partner Relational Problem:* a label given to patients when there is "a pattern of interaction between spouses or partners characterized by negative communication (e.g., criticisms), distorted communication (e.g., unrealistic expectations), or noncommunication (e.g., withdrawal) that is associated with clinically significant impairment in individual or family functioning or the development of symptoms in one or both partners." (In other words, a normal marriage during a bad week.)
- *Identity Problem:* used "when the focus of clinical attention is uncertainty about multiple issues relating to identity such as long-term goals, career choice, friendship patterns, sexual orientation and behavior, moral values, and group loyalties." (In other words, normal young adulthood—or "midlife crisis.")
- *Phase-of-Life Problem:* used to label "problems associated with entering school, leaving parental control, starting a new career, and changes involved in marriage, divorce, and retirement." (In other words, normal everyday life.)

Including these categories as DSM "diagnoses" is a serious semantic error because a diagnosis implies that there is a disease or disorder to begin with. It implies that any individual experiencing negative emotions in response to a life situation is abnormal, and that his or her problems are pathological rather than simply a natural part of living. But there is nothing pathological about a critical husband, a wife with unrealistic expectations, a college student uncertain about "leaving parental control," or anyone unsure about career choices or "group loyalties." If we weren't occasionally confused, argumentative, critical, worried, or frightened, we wouldn't be human. Choices, mistakes, and growth are part of life.

Even more problems arise when normal behavioral variants and eccentricities—shyness, a melodramatic personality, conceitedness, dependency—are labeled as personality "disorders": avoidant personality disorder, histrionic personality disorder, narcissism, dependent personality disorder. Once a patient receives such a label, a therapist is likely to try talking him or her into undergoing lengthy and expensive therapy (and taking medications such as Prozac).

Yet much of what makes us interesting as human beings is our differences and eccentricities; where would Madonna be, for instance, without her "histrionic" personality? Probably working as a grocery checker in Queens, hiding her underwear safely under her apron. And Bill Gates, shorn of his eccentric personality traits, would probably be just another computer engineer—and not the world's wealthiest software developer. Albert Einstein, Thomas Edison, Charles Darwin, Wolfgang Amadeus Mozart, and Abraham Lincoln all were, by modern psychiatry's definition, troubled people in need of "help." In fact, most of our great artists, musicians, entrepreneurs, and actors have personalities the DSM would define as pathological—and, in most cases, those personality traits are largely responsible for their success. "There's a place for different personalities because there are different paths in life," psychologist Carol Eagle says. "We shouldn't pathologize difference."

Unfortunately, psychiatry often does just that, particularly when dealing with female patients. A number of studies have shown that psychiatrists are more apt to prescribe extensive therapy for women's minor personality quirks than for men's, suggesting that longtime psychoanalytic stereotypes about women being naturally unstable and mentally unhealthy are still alive and well. Caplan, noticing that many of DSM's categories and proposed categories (premenstrual dysphoric disorder, self-defeating personality disorder, and so on) attempt to pathologize normal aspects of being female, and that few of the categories characterize common male behaviors such as competitiveness and aggressiveness as abnormal, once gave a talk entitled, "Do Mental Health Professionals Think There Is a Normal Woman?"

Psychiatry also is unwittingly influenced by what researcher Martin L. Gross calls "emotional fashion." As Gross points out in *The Psychological Society,* "A woman raised in Victorian England who was sexually inhibited would be considered emotionally normal. The same type of woman, suffering from sexual anxiety in the late 1970s, would soon find herself in psychotherapy for her 'neurosis.'" The term "neurosis" itself went out of fashion a few years ago, so now the same woman would probably be labeled as having "anxiety disorder"—or perhaps "sexual disorder not otherwise specified"—and would be given both psychotherapy *and* Prozac! Similarly, fervent religious devotion—once an almost universal characteristic—is now considered suspect by many therapists. Conversely, promiscuity, which previous generations of psychiatrists would have considered pathological, became "normal" during the sexual revolution of the 1960s. And at one early point in psychiatry's history, slaves brave enough to escape captivity were labeled as having a psychiatric disorder called "drapetomania," because their behavior struck doctors as mentally unbalanced! In short, people whose behavior and temperament are out of sync with societal norms are likely to be labeled as "disturbed," and people whose behavior fits the current norms are likely to be considered "normal." Thus, many perfectly normal people are labeled as ill simply because they have out-of-fashion personalities.

Personality variations such as timidness, boldness, dependency, or assertiveness—whether they occur in men or in women—are not signs of a "mental disorder," and labeling them that way can seriously affect an individual's outlook and self-confidence. Remember: there is nothing abnormal about minor life problems, personality variations, and minor eccentricities—and none of them requires prolonged, expensive therapy. Don't let a therapist convince you that you're suffering from a "pathological" personality if all you want is help with a few personal problems.

A Caveat: The Therapist Is Not a God

Although many therapists bill themselves as experts on the human psyche, most of them don't know any more about it than you do. And this is every bit as true of the psychiatrist with advanced psychoanalytic training as it is of the non-M.D. therapist.

This is hard for Americans to accept, because of our ingrained stereotype of psychiatrists as all-knowing "mind doctors" (a stereotype exemplified by the recent miniseries, *Op Center,* in which a government psychiatrist is described as "our official mind-reader and Good Witch of the East. . . . Tell her how a man behaves, she'll tell you what he's thinking and what he's going to do next."). We believe that psychiatrists, in addition to understanding how our brains work, can understand our "minds." We believe that psychiatrists are somehow able to know what we're thinking, what we're feeling, and what we're *planning* to think and feel and do—that, in short, they know us better than we know ourselves. We envision them as mental super-beings, able to see into our most secret thoughts and emotions as easily as Superman sees through walls. (It's rumored, for instance, that Richard Nixon would not allow psychiatrists in the room with him, for fear that they could somehow read his thoughts—and that reclusive millionaire Howard Hughes avoided them for the same reason.)

"As experts on mental disease," Jerrold Maxmen comments, in *The New Psychiatry,* "psychiatrists are supposed to be experts on *all thinking, feeling, and behaving.* But since every human endeavor involves thinking, feeling, and behaving, psychiatrists are widely assumed to have *unique insights into absolutely everything—* the most obvious area being mental health."

This assumption, to anyone who knows psychiatrists, is pretty funny. As Maxmen points out, "being ordinary people, shrinks don't know anything more about finding happiness than anyone else." In fact, they may know far less: studies show that rates of suicide and drug addiction are significantly higher among psychiatrists than among the general population or among practitioners in other stressful medical professions. According to at least one study, psychiatrists also are more likely than other people to have family histories of mental illness. Swiss researchers studying military records found that psychiatrists were vastly more likely than surgeons or internists to have been rejected for military service on grounds of "mental" disorders. And anyone who has attended a conference of psychiatrists can tell you that their interpersonal skills could use improvement!

It's been suggested, in fact, that psychiatrists go into the profession largely to find out what's wrong with their own personalities. (In one survey, 25 percent of 531 psychiatrists said they chose the field because of their own psychiatric problems or treatment.) If so, there's little evidence that they've benefited from their choice of career. Although there are many exceptions, both patients and other doctors say they find psychiatrists as a group to be aloof, supercilious, and somewhat odd. It's ironic that the profession most interested in delving into people's feelings and motivations seems to attract more eccentric practitioners than any other medical field.

I'm not trying to belittle psychiatrists (after all, I am one myself); I'm merely pointing out that they're not superhuman or infallible—a very important fact to keep in mind if you decide to participate in psychotherapy. Remember that psychiatrists can suggest possible causes of your problems, and help you seek solutions, but they won't always be right because they have no magic insight into what makes people tick. Often, in fact, they have no personal experience at all in the area of mental health in which they consider themselves "experts." (An acquaintance of mine once conducted a lengthy news interview with a child psychiatrist who offered readers authoritative advice on everything from bedwetting to handling homework problems. At the end of the interview, the psychiatrist—who spent most of his time conducting therapy sessions for parents of young children—admitted that he had little firsthand experience with children outside the office, had no children himself, and didn't intend to have any!)

So don't take everything your therapist says as the gospel truth. As Caplan cautions, in *They Say You're Crazy,* "[Therapists] are human beings. Some of them grew up in your neighborhood. Some got lower grades than you did in high school. Some graduated at the bottom of the programs in which they learned to 'treat' you, but you will never know that from the certificates on their walls." As in any profession, there are good and bad practitioners, experienced and inexperienced practitioners, caring and apathetic practitioners, and smart and ignorant practitioners.

Furthermore, psychotherapy is a subjective process, and every therapist brings his or her own biases, weaknesses, and moral/political/social baggage to the therapy session. A feminist therapist may blame a female patient's problems on an oppressive husband, while a classically trained Freudian analyst may blame exactly the same problems on the woman's deep-rooted attraction to her father. A therapist who believes emotional symptoms are caused by repressed memories will find such memories in nearly every patient. And therapists—who tend to be liberal, sexually "progressive," and agnostic or nonpracticing when it comes to religion—often have preconceived negative ideas about the mental health of patients who are religious, conservative, or just plain modest. The old adage, "You see what you look for," was never more true than in psychotherapy!

It's also true that you *don't* see what you *don't* look for—which generally means that patients with physical illnesses will get short shrift from psychotherapists. Healy notes:

> Many depressed patients repeatedly tell their therapists that there is no reason for their loss of interest or their loss of energy. . . . That what they feel is something different [from] sadness and unhappiness and much more like something physical. We typically ignore or even fail to hear them say this. . . . Paradoxically, this is most likely to be the case in psychiatry of all medical specialties, even though it, more than any other specialty, seemingly pays heed to what patients say."

Remember that the psychotherapist is, in most cases, neither trained to look for physical disease nor philosophically inclined to consider it as a possibility. (In fact, most therapists prefer to treat only patients they consider as "psychologically sophisticated"—a fancy way of saying patients willing to believe that their problems are all "mental" rather than physical.)

The Bottom Line

Therapy can help a patient deal with the emotional complications that naturally occur when he or she suffers from brain dysfunction, but it can't cure the dysfunction itself. And therapy can help a person with "problems in living," but only if it doesn't create problems where none exist.

Most importantly, therapy is not a medical treatment. Therefore, it's a tool to be used *only* after a patient undergoes a careful deductive differential evaluation and receives a diagnosis—not a DSM label, but a real diagnosis—and medical intervention, if necessary. A patient with significant behavioral symptoms who is given a DSM label and referred for psychotherapy without being thoroughly evaluated for physical illness is, in my opinion, a victim of medical mistreatment.

So, too, is a patient referred for therapy by a psychiatrist who hasn't carefully investigated the techniques and professionalism of the therapist being recommended. This scenario is all too common: a psychiatrist refers patients to a therapist who's a social acquaintance or relative, or who has an office down the hall, without checking to see what methods the therapist uses and what therapeutic philosophies he or she subscribes to. Such referrals can be dangerous: not all therapy helps, and some therapy harms. In fact, as we'll see in the next chapter, many patients are being permanently injured by current "pop psychiatry" therapies based on faulty and dangerous practices.

CHAPTER 6

Talk Soup Can Make You Sick

As long as practitioners are not accountable for what they lead their clients to believe and what they encourage them to do, they will remain reckless.

Richard Ofshe and Ethan Watters
in "Making Monsters," *Society* Magazine

P SYCHIATRIST JOHN MACK, A HARVARD MEDICAL SCHOOL professor, appeared on the *Oprah Winfrey Show* not long ago to tell about his current work: conducting hypnotherapy sessions for patients who have been abducted by aliens from outer space. Although Mack is coy about whether he believes in alien visits himself, he assures his patients that their experiences are normal, and that their kidnappers are well-meaning types who are visiting our planet only to keep us from self-destructing. He knows all of this, of course, because he's a psychiatrist.

Psychiatry is big business these days for Mack and other psychiatrists making the talk show rounds. If you watch TV talk shows on a regular basis, odds are you've heard psychiatrists talk about the wonders of Prozac and Ritalin. You've heard about treating your "psychospiritual crisis" and freeing your inner child. You've heard that your mental problems are caused by cold and aloof parents, "smothering" parents, unresponsive spouses, a lack of self-esteem, or an uncaring society. And, of course, you've heard about the aliens.

Unfortunately, what you haven't heard about is the real science of psychiatry. When is the last time you heard a psychiatrist telling a talk show audience how he cured a hyperactive child after finding parasites in his stool sample? Or treated a suicidally despondent woman by curing her thyroid imbalance? The media thrive on the new and exciting, so you're not going to hear very often about the psychiatrists (and there are a number of them) who cure their patients the old-fashioned way: by diagnosing and treating what's wrong with them. The more logical and scientifically grounded a treatment is, the less newsworthy the media consider it. Conversely, the more bizarre a doctor's claims are, the more likely that he or she will appear on the talk shows or get headlines in the papers. The farther psychiatry strays from medical science the more popular it becomes with the media, because Prozac and psychobabble are much easier to discuss—and more entertaining— than malfunctioning brain cells.

A Plethora of Kooks

There are plenty of far-out practitioners for the media to cover. All fields of medicine have their pop practitioners, but psychiatry has been overrun by them. Why? Because DSM, by popularizing meaningless "diagnoses" such as "phase of life problem" or "parent–child relational problem," has reinforced the idea that a catchy label is equivalent to a diagnosis. Furthermore, DSM has refused to take a stand regarding the causes and proper treatment of brain dysfunction. Thus, the door has been opened for a slew of nonsensical therapies. (After all, if any label can be a diagnosis, and there are no correct or incorrect treatment procedures, anything goes.) Pop practitioners, from alien abduction therapists to computer con artists who promise to "diagnose schizophrenia in two minutes," are doing a land-office business. And why not? The process of devolution from pseudoscience to new age mysticism or computerized "diagnosis" is only natural: it's a short step, after all, from nondiagnostic DSM-IV labels such as "identity problem" to pop psychiatry's "psychospiritual crisis," or a two-minute diagnosis of schizophrenia offered by a floppy disk.

The concept of cookbook symptom lists, popularized by DSM, also lends itself well to pop psychiatry. Mack, for instance, offers a list of the most common symptoms of alien abduction: fear of the dark, repetitive nightmares, dreams about abduction, phobias or fears, and the appearance of unexplained scars, cuts, or bruises. Imagine: with only this simple list of five symptoms, you are now qualified to "diagnose" abduction by aliens! (A potentially lucrative practice, as some "experts" in the psychiatric effects of alien abduction estimate that more than 3 million of us have been abducted.) Mack's list, silly as it is, is a natural outgrowth of DSM's diagnosis-by-checklist mentality.

It's not just pop psychiatry that DSM encourages, but pop psychology as well. That's because DSM, although ostensibly a "diagnostic" manual for psychiatric MDs, states up front that it's also designed for psychologists, counselors, and other health and mental health professionals. In other words, DSM is allegedly a book on how to make medical diagnoses, but heck, you don't even need a degree in medicine to use it. Thus, a non-M.D. therapist— a psychologist or social worker, for instance—can "diagnose" patients by using DSM, and can offer any sort of psychotherapy for patients' perceived disorders. As a result, hundreds of pop psychology therapies—primal scream, rebirthing, Rolfing, codependency therapies—are being pushed for patients labeled as depressed, anxious, or troubled.

Medical practitioners in other fields are generally outspoken about approaches they find unscientific or dangerous—thus squelching media enthusiasm over them—but psychiatrists tend to remain quiet about silly treatments such as primal scream and alien abduction therapy. And psychiatry appears to have no objection when psychologists, social workers, and other lay practitioners usurp its role by "diagnosing" patients via the DSM and "treating" them with pop therapies. Why don't psychiatrists object? Because they have strayed so far from proper medical diagnosis and treatment themselves that they are in no position to criticize those who have gone a few steps further. Of all the medical fields, psychiatry has been the most open to bizarre treatments and the least amenable to scientific investigation and verification.

The upshot is that the public is highly vulnerable to exploitation by pop psychiatrists and pop psychologists, who are generally either protected or ignored by their mainstream colleagues. "The professions involved [psychiatry and psychology] are too immature to have developed viable procedures for restraining excesses," say sociologists Richard Ofshe and Ethan Watters, "and have no way of prohibiting rank experimentation with humans."

Much pop psychiatry and pop psychology is harmless stuff. If you want to believe that your mate has a Tinkerbell complex, or you want to stand in a room and scream at the top of your lungs, it probably won't hurt you—*if* there's nothing wrong with you in the first place. But any pop therapies can be dangerous to patients who *do* suffer from serious brain dysfunction, and who turn to such therapies instead of obtaining a real diagnosis and appropriate intervention. For patients with progressive diseases, a year in primal scream therapy can literally be fatal.

Although many pop psychiatry and pop psychology fads are simply foolish, several current fads have particular potential to cause devastating harm to psychiatric patients and their families. Some of the most destructive fads warrant a close look.

Fad 1. "Toxic Parent" Therapies

Talk shows regularly feature psychiatrists who explain why John suffers from anxiety (his father was overprotective), why Jane abuses drugs (her parents subconsciously rejected her), or why Tom is a mass murderer (his father was cold and unfeeling—or perhaps overly affectionate and threatening). The most popular theme of pop psychiatry is also the oldest theme of Freudian psychiatry: whatever is wrong with you is all your mother's (or sometimes your father's) fault. What's more, according to many psychiatrists, even the most minor of parental faults—cutting the apron strings too late, assigning too many chores, or attending too few Little League games—can lead to disastrous consequences.

One of the chief figures in the blame-your-parents school of psychiatry is Peter Breggin, author of *Toxic Psychiatry* and *Talking Back to Prozac*—best-selling books that are usually prominently displayed in the medical sections of bookstores. Breggin, to his credit, attacks the wholesale use of psychotropic drugs, but his own treatments for "mental" illness are equally misguided and potentially life-threatening.

Breggin argues that most psychiatric disorders have no biological roots whatsoever; in fact, the index of *Toxic Psychiatry* doesn't contain even one listing for "diagnosis." Instead, Breggin claims that many psychiatric symptoms stem from "toxic parenting," alleging that psychiatric patients—or, as he calls them, people undergoing "psychospiritual crises"—have suffered childhood traumas that left them irrevocably scarred. (These traumas, according to his book, may be as subtle as "negative vibrations" from parents.) He does charitably allow that "not all families with children in spiritual despair are obviously abusive," but he adds, in the same breath, that "there is almost always a severe psychospiritual incompatibility between the labeled patient and one or both parents." (Note the use of the term "labeled," insinuating that the family members of a psychiatric patient are as disturbed as the patient, and simply haven't yet been identified as "patients" themselves.)

In other words, Breggin blames virtually all serious psychiatric disorders on bad parents—not just the kind of parents who beat their children or sell them to strangers for cocaine, but also the kind of parents who occasionally project "bad vibes." He's not the only psychiatrist to do this: Paula Caplan and Ian Hall-McCorquodale note, in "Mother-Blaming in Major Clinical Journals," that parents—particularly mothers—have been blamed for bad dreams, tantrums, truancy, chronic vomiting, arson, poor concentration, sleepwalking, and even ulcerative colitis. But Breggin has perhaps done more than any other professional since Bruno Bettelheim (who accused both "refrigerator mothers" and "smother mothers" of causing psychosis) to promote the parents-cause-mental-illness theory.

It's a wonderful theory from the media's point of view: it's simple to explain, easily believed by the public, and conducive to an endless stream of talk shows featuring angry, screaming children and defensive, crying parents. But, whether it raises TV ratings or not, it's baloney.

In the first place, there is no evidence linking serious mental illness to bad parenting. Three decades ago, during the heyday of psychoanalytic psychiatry and psychology, psychologist George Frank reviewed the scientific literature and came to a conclusion that has been proven valid by virtually every study that followed:

> Psychologists have reasoned that the experiences the individual has in his early life at home . . . are major determinants in . . . the development of psychopathology. A review of the research of the past 40 years failed to support this assumption. No factors were found in the parent–child interaction of schizophrenics, neurotics or those with behavior disorders which could be identified as unique to them or which could distinguish one group from the other, or any of the groups from the families of the controls. [Frank, *Psychological Bulletin*]

Psychologist Arlene Skolnick, an expert on child development, has noted in *Psychology Today* that "most children who experience disorder and early sorrow grow up to be adequate adults. Further, studies sampling 'normal' or 'superior' people—college students, business executives, professionals, creative artists, and scientists—find such 'pathological' conditions in similar or greater proportions. Thus, many studies trying to document the effects of early pathological and traumatic conditions have failed to demonstrate more than a weak link between them and later development."

Among the studies supporting Skolnick's claim was one commissioned years before by the U.S. Air Force, and reported by H. Renaud and F. Estess. The subjects were 100 exceptional Air Force officers who excelled both on the job and in their personal lives. Researchers assumed their data would show that these men came from wonderful, caring, nurturing families; they were amazed to find, on the contrary, that their happy group of achievers came from family settings as "pathological" as those of the researchers' psychiatric patients. In another study cited by E. Fuller Torrey, in *The Death of Psychiatry,* experienced psychiatrists, psychiatric residents, and people off the street were asked to examine the life experiences of 34 individuals, and then to predict what "mental" problems they might be suffering in adulthood as a result. None of the three groups was able to predict, based on the subjects' early histories, whether they'd grown up to be neurotic, psychotic, or just plain normal. The author of this study concluded that the data "clearly challenge the idea that it is meaningful to discuss specific life experiences as predisposing to a given illness."

One other classic study, by Jean Macfarlane and her colleagues, followed 200 children from infancy through adolescence, and then reevaluated them at age 30. The researchers assumed that the children from troubled homes would have serious problems as adults, and that the children from happy homes would be well adjusted. Surprise! The researchers were startled to find that *two-thirds of their predictions were wrong.* Children from troubled homes often did extremely well as adults, while many children from good homes—particularly boys who were stars on their athletic teams, and girls who were beautiful and popular in high school—had difficulty coping in adulthood.

Dozens of similar studies have shown that, except in cases of extreme abuse or neglect, there's little connection between people's early upbringing and their emotional health in later life. Conversely, there is a wealth of evidence linking psychiatric disorders to brain dysfunction. Regarding behavioral disorders—particularly those categorized as psychoses—the nature–nurture debate has been conclusively decided in favor of nature.

Take autism as an example. This syndrome—made famous by Dustin Hoffman's Oscar-winning performance as an autistic savant in *Rainman*—affects thousands of children and adults in the

United States. The term "autism" is not a diagnosis, but a label for an odd collection of severely disabling symptoms—aloofness, lack of language (or poor language skills), resistance to change, a lack of pretending skills, odd behaviors such as hand-flapping, and abnormal reactions to sights, sounds, and touch. The syndrome occurs at similar rates across different countries, cultures, and ethnic groups. Some children labeled as autistic have remarkable savant skills—singing arias in infancy, playing sonatas by ear, and performing complex mathematical calculations in seconds. Yet most autistic individuals (including the savants) remain severely disabled throughout their lives, and even those who outgrow many of their symptoms are usually somewhat peculiar.

Here's what we know about autism so far. Most children labeled as autistic are retarded, and about one-third have seizures. Both autopsy studies and brain scans of living subjects have linked autism to brain abnormalities (usually underdevelopment of the cerebellum, an area at the back of the brain). Autistic symptoms can be caused by metabolic disorders and by prenatal viruses such as rubella. (Rubella in adolescence and adulthood can also, in rare cases, cause autism: several cases have been reported in which perfectly normal, healthy, happy individuals, within days of contracting rubella, developed severe, permanent symptoms of autism.) Biochemical studies show that levels of brain "messenger" chemicals are abnormal in autistic children, and twin studies—used to compare the influence of nature and nurture—clearly indicate that many cases of autism are genetically determined. In short, researchers consider the evidence of autism's biological roots to be overwhelming. In fact, the problem researchers now face is that they have discovered so many—not so few—biological abnormalities in autistic subjects.

Still, Breggin blames autistic symptoms on parents who show children "little warmth or attention!" This outdated theory, first dreamed up by psychologist Bruno Bettelheim decades ago, was abandoned by researchers in the late 1960s after scientific studies showed that it was false. Breggin's determination to resurrect this dead theory, in the face of a mountain of evidence contradicting it, shows a blatant disregard for—or complete ignorance of—the facts.

Similarly, Breggin ignores a vast body of evidence linking schizophrenia to genetic vulnerability, prenatal viral infections, toxic exposure, and brain defects, and accuses schizophrenics' families of somehow causing or exacerbating their disorder by "frustrating their progress toward selfhood." He claims that depression is the fault of guilt-provoking parents, who raise children "caught between the pursuit of their own chosen adult values and those taught to them as children by their religious, educational, and family institutions." And he recently blamed hyperactive behavior on parents who "are unable, ill-equipped, or unwilling to raise children in a secure, disciplined and loving manner," and on schools that "fail to respond to the moral, social and educational needs of youngsters." Never mind that there is not a single shred of scientific evidence to support any of these charges.

But then, scientific evidence is not Breggin's forte; in fact, he complains that "as long as we consider psychiatry a 'science,' it will seem odd to go back in time to an era when the basic principles, if not the practices, often surpassed our own." The only practices Breggin seems to endorse, however, are "love and compassion," which have never—in any era—cured syphilis, tumors, endocrine dysfunction, meningitis, or other disorders affecting the brain. Furthermore, it's difficult to understand how a doctor who ignores the biological roots of behavioral and emotional disorders—thereby potentially endangering the lives and sanity of his patients—can be more loving or compassionate than a doctor who successfully diagnoses, treats, and cures his patients. And it's hard to understand how Breggin, a psychiatrist who prides himself on being compassionate, can lay such terrible guilt on parents who have played no role—except, in some cases, an unwitting genetic one—in causing their children's tragic disorders.

The blame placed on these parents by doctors like Breggin often is crushing. One couple I know, the parents of a child with

Tourette's syndrome, spent years (and thousands of dollars) undergoing therapy in an attempt to discover how they had caused their child's obsessive-compulsive behavior—only to learn, when the child was finally diagnosed, that such behavior is a well-documented symptom of this genetic disorder. Another couple, the adoptive parents of two children with fetal alcohol syndrome, were blamed for decades by psychoanalysts for their children's academic and social failings—failings which actually stemmed from serious brain dysfunction due to prenatal damage. Perhaps Breggin would benefit from talking to families like these, whose lives, already made difficult by their children's problems, were further burdened by "blame therapies" that did nothing to help their children.

Why is Breggin so popular, despite his archaic and unscientific views? Because few psychiatrists dare to speak out against his approaches, at least in public. DSM, after all, encourages psychiatrists to be nonjudgmental about different viewpoints and therapies, no matter how little evidence there is to support them. By refusing to state categorically that "mental" disorders are brain disorders, DSM allows practitioners to blame any causes at all—including parental "bad vibes"—for brain dysfunction.

Fad 2. Repressed Memory Therapy and Other "Blame Games"

Breggin and generations of other psychoanalytic psychiatrists have spawned dozens of pop psychiatry and pop psychology offshoots, all based on the premise that diagnosis is unnecessary because all "mental" illness results from childhood trauma. Prominent among these offshoots is repressed memory therapy, in which troubled adults supposedly become well again after dealing with previously buried memories of sexual abuse, physical violence, or even Satanic rituals. (A remarkable number of suburban housewives in the 1950s and 1960s seem to have practiced Satan worship!) In the early 1990s, repressed memory therapy became a popular therapy for patients—primarily women—labeled by DSM as having borderline personality, depression, post-traumatic stress disorder, eating disorders, and dysthymic disorder.

Repressed memory therapy begins with convincing a patient that some form of abuse actually occurred—even if the patient has absolutely no recall of such an event. "What starts as a guess about what type of abuse might have caused their present emotional problems," Ofshe and Watters say in a *Society* article aptly entitled "Making Monsters," "grows into guessing which relative committed the abuse. Repetitive retelling and reshaping of this account can transform a 'perhaps' into a 'for sure' and can thereby create a sense of certainty. The process may culminate in elaborate fantasies about schemes by parents, neighbors, teachers, or any other adults who were around during the client's childhood." A large percentage of patients also become convinced, with the help of their therapists, that they have multiple personalities, some of which have repressed their memories.

The big problem with repressed memory therapy is that, in almost all cases that have been scientifically evaluated, the memories are not repressed but completely false. A 1995 study by Harrison Pope and James Hudson, in *Psychological Medicine*, reports that "laboratory studies over the past 60 years have failed to demonstrate that individuals can 'repress' memories;" conversely, there is considerable evidence that persuasive therapists can cause patients to create false memories of events that never happened, including memories of molestation, abuse, and Satan worship. Researcher Elizabeth Loftus, an expert on memory, says that the entire concept of repressed memories is seriously flawed. "[M]emory surprises me again and again with its gee-whiz gullibility," she says in her book, *The Myth of Repressed Memory,* adding that she has been able to "implant false memories in people's minds, making them believe in characters who never existed and events that never happened."

All of the evidence to date clearly indicates that the overwhelming majority of "repressed memory" patients are simply brainwashed into believing in the reality of totally fictitious events. Furthermore, virtually all patients undergoing repressed memory therapy appear to get worse, not better. Even patients who originally entered repressed memory therapy with relatively minor problems frequently wind up bitter, withdrawn, distrustful, and emotionally devastated. Loftus, writing about a group of five women who underwent repressed memory therapy, says one had a mental breakdown, one tried to commit suicide, and one nearly destroyed her marriage—and "four of the five women were given drugs to relieve their depression, rage, anxiety and suicidal tendencies."

"Let's even assume that [repressed memories] are real; they're all true," psychologist Chris Barden told an *Insight* reporter. "Even with that assumption, this type of therapy makes patients worse than they were! Who is it helping?"

Almost no one, apparently—yet the repressed memory movement has caught fire in America. Thousands of books have been sold by repressed memory therapist Renee Fredrickson, who claims that a history of repressed memories of sexual abuse "lurks in the background of millions of ordinary, high functioning Americans." Other therapists have written books and articles linking symptoms such as irritable bowel syndrome, PMS, obesity, and dating problems to repressed memories. And celebrities, always an easy mark for new therapies, have climbed on the bandwagon: actress Roseanne Barr, for instance, reportedly claims to remember her mother molesting her while changing her diaper.

It's true that most repressed memory therapy sessions are conducted by psychologists (although a number of psychiatrists also practice the technique), and that some psychiatrists have come forward to condemn repressed memory therapy, as the evidence mounts that it is not therapy but blatant brainwashing and manipulation. Yet, as Ofshe and Watters note, "Legitimation of recovered memory theory by academia is contributing to the institutionalization of the therapy," which is now being taught in some psychiatric residency programs, promoted in psychiatric workshops and seminars, and practiced in a number of psychiatric hospitals. It is hard to imagine another field of medicine taking so quickly to a treatment that virtually all evidence reveals to be quackery, and making it part of its mainstream philosophy. (One wonders when DSM will make it a diagnosis.)

Many of the patients receiving repressed memory therapy are referred by psychiatrists who base their referrals on DSM labels. And most of these psychiatrists fail to follow up to ensure that the therapies they've recommended are helping rather than hurting their patients. The fact that most psychiatrists refer patients to nonpsychiatric therapists, rather than conduct therapy themselves, does not absolve them of responsibility for the consequences of ineffective or harmful therapeutic techniques.

These consequences have been tragic for thousands of families. Relationships have been irretrievably ruined, careers and marriages ended, fortunes spent on legal defense, and jail terms served by innocent family members convicted of crimes that never occurred. These cases are not isolated incidents; the False Memory Syndrome Foundation, composed primarily of people who say they have been unjustly accused of abuse or molestation after relatives received repressed memory therapy, had 4,600 members by 1993. Equally devastated are the patients themselves: torn away from their families, told that their childhoods were lies and their relationships were frauds, few are able to put their lives back together again. Ofshe says therapists have subjected repressed memory patients to "the closest thing to the experience of rape and brutalization that can ever be done without actually touching them." None of this appears to bother repressed memory therapists; Fredrickson, for instance, says airily that "if months or years down the road you find you are mistaken about details, you can always apologize and set the record straight." Not likely, if mom has committed suicide and dad's still in jail.

Repressed memory therapy is only one of dozens of parent-blaming therapies. One of the best known is primal scream therapy, developed by psychologist Arthur Janov in the late 1950s and still used by a number of therapists. The therapy consists of making patients lie spread-eagled on the therapist's floor and talk about how terrible their lives have been, for hours and hours, until they finally scream out something like, "Mommy, I hate you!" After about a year of this, Janov says, patients have advanced so much that they can scream by themselves at home.

More recent are codependency and recovery therapies, which also generally blame the parents of "victims" for all of their emotional and behavioral problems. The titles of major books on codependency and recovery—*Forgiving Your Parents, Toxic Parents,* and *Divorcing a Parent*—are a good indication of what they preach, which is that every adult is a small, helpless child unable to grow into adulthood because of parental neglect, abuse, or—as Breggin would say—"bad vibrations."

Reading such books, one wonders if it's at all possible to raise a "normal" child. Consider this partial list of danger signs, taken from *Kids Who Carry Our Pain*, by Robert Hemfelt and Paul Warren (bearing in mind that answering "yes" to even a few questions means you're dysfunctional):

> "Are there more than one or two evening meals per week at which the entire family is not gathered?"
> "Do you and your spouse promise over and over to spend more time—better time—with each other and the kids? Are such promises frequently broken?"
> "Does the level of 'busyness' remain high in your household?"
> "Do you find yourself doubting frequently that you really know your children?"

Even this short list would cover virtually all parents of teenagers (has anyone ever really known a teenager?!), all families with two working parents, and all families with regular outside activities in the evening. Thus, if you're a working woman, or the parent of a 16-year-old going through normal adolescent moodiness and angst, or a father who volunteers with the fire department two nights a week, your family is broken and your child needs therapy.

Most codependency therapy participants, however, are not children but adults still suffering—supposedly—from long-term wounds caused by neglectful, distant, or thoughtless parents. Participants in codependency and recovery therapies spend hours writing letters to their "wounded inner children," conduct "divorce rituals" over their deceased parents' graves, and perform dozens of other "healing" exercises. They estimate their "codependency scores," write down their feelings on an hour-by-hour basis, and draw family trees to chart past generations of abuse. The end result, generally, is not healing but a morbid preoccupation with tiny slights and insults that happened decades (or even generations) ago.

Therapist Frank Pittman III, a critic of such "victim" therapies, charges, in *Psychology Today,* that they encourage patients to "resign from the adult world, eschew responsibility for their conduct in relationships, and whimper that the world owes them a life." He adds that "the victim identity is like a doctor's excuse from a gym class or history exam, only it is an excuse from life itself." Psychiatrist E. Fuller Torrey, in an even harsher assessment of parent-blaming therapies, says that "in the areas of child-rearing, mental health, and criminal justice, the denial of personal responsibility has had a grimly unhumanistic effect.

"[T]he corollary to don't-blame-me is blame-my-parents," he told the *Washington Monthly.* "In the Freudian schema, mother, father, family, social circumstance, and culture become the causal agents for whatever is wrong. The ripple of personal irresponsibility spreads outward until the very terms 'good' and 'bad' seem to lose their meaning."

Steven Wolin, another of the handful of psychiatrists willing to criticize victim therapies, says they are based on the "damage" model, which he calls a "prophecy of doom." Such a model, Wolin believes, is inappropriate even for people whose families did have serious problems. "It basically says," Wolin told a *Psychology Today* interviewer, "that if your family is having trouble, the chances that you are going to [experience problems] are very high. It derives from traditional psychiatric thinking, conventional wisdom, and popular psychology, which stress how children growing up in adverse circumstances suffer lasting emotional disturbances." Wolin, noting that most children from troubled families are able to survive and thrive, calls on therapists to replace the damage model with a resiliency model. "We are filled with a vocabulary of pathology," he says. "There is no *Diagnostic and Statistical Manual* for strengths."

Even when serious abuse has occurred—as in the case of victims of incest—survivors have much more trouble recovering and getting on with their lives when their therapy focuses only on the trauma itself, rather than acknowledging participants' strengths, interests, and future goals. I'm not saying that people shouldn't talk about traumatic experiences; patients who have been raped, or molested, or abused often need a safe and understanding listener to whom they can unburden themselves and express their anger and pain. But after that's done, the therapist should ask: "Where do you go from here?" Chronic, never-ending victimhood is corrosive; overcoming a trauma and moving forward is liberating. (There is some evidence, fortunately, that therapists themselves are beginning to see the dangers of blame therapy. When Wolin spoke at a recent conference for 4,000 therapists, telling them that they were helping to turn America into "a nation of emotional cripples," he received a standing ovation.)

"Blame therapy" practitioners will *tell* you, of course, that their approaches are liberating and healing. However, few such therapists subject their patient data to rigorous analysis—the only meaningful way to tell whether a treatment is effective. That's because these therapies can't be demonstrated to be effective, and because they *can* be demonstrated to be "toxic" to many patients.

Parent-blaming therapies destroy patients' families. They create enormous guilt in innocent parties. They offer excuses for maladaptive behavior, which tends to exacerbate behavior problems (witness the Hollywood celebrities whose behavior becomes more aberrant after each therapy they undergo).

Even more importantly, therapists who blame every behavioral disorder on childhood trauma *aren't going to diagnose* psychiatric patients suffering from serious, treatable disorders. For instance, a section on assessing childhood problems, in the codependency book *Kids Who Carry Our Pain*, asks, "Has one or more of your children been diagnosed as hyperactive?" and "Does your child suffer persistent or chronic physical health problems not explained by medical work-ups?" If so, the book says, "quite probably trouble lies ahead for your family." Well, indeed it does, if you attempt to treat hyperactivity and other persistent medical problems with codependency therapy instead of finding their causes and correcting them.

Fad 3. Media-Hyped "Wonder Drugs"

Drug therapy is a mainstream psychiatric approach, but the media frequently create "pop" drugs. In fact, the media are as effective at starting drug fads as they are at starting fashion fads. Within days of a major TV or magazine story on a new miracle drug, doctors' offices are jammed with patients clamoring for it, and sales go through the roof.

As I've already mentioned, Peter Kramer's *Listening to Prozac*—promoted by hundreds of newspaper articles and TV interviews—has helped push sales of Prozac into the millions. Unfortunately, Kramer is only one of dozens of psychiatrists and psychologists making the rounds of talk shows to promote the use of psychotropic drugs for an ever-expanding list of DSM "diagnoses." For instance, Dr. James Goodwin (nicknamed "Doctor Feelgood") has appeared on *Oprah*, *Good Morning America*, and the

BBC, promoting Prozac for people with low self-esteem, chronic irritability, eating problems, hypersexuality, and virtually every other mental symptom it's possible to experience. Goodwin claims, in fact, that three-quarters of the population would benefit from Prozac. And Prozac isn't the only drug getting massive promotion from the media; *Time*'s recent cover story on "adult hyperactivity" sent thousands of readers to their doctors seeking prescriptions for Ritalin.

The media are quick to react each time a mind-altering "miracle drug" arrives on the scene. Before adequate studies can verify initial results, hundreds of media reports are published, and thousands (or even millions) of desperate patients obtain prescriptions. Unfortunately, virtually all drugs are later found to have serious shortcomings or side effects. These later reports, however, rarely make it out of the medical journals and onto the front pages.

An important rule of thumb lay readers should keep in mind, when reading about new "wonder drugs," is that *early reports almost always inflate the benefits, and underestimate the risks, of new drugs*. That's because initial reports are much more dramatic and newsworthy than the research that follows. Positive studies almost always generate interest; negative studies tend to be ignored.

Fenfluramine, a drug that alters levels of the brain chemical serotonin, is a good example. This amphetamine-like drug, originally prescribed for dieters, was tested, in 1982, on three autistic children, in a study with no control subjects. Despite the study's shortcomings, its positive results were reported in the *New England Journal of Medicine*. That same week, headlines began appearing in major papers: "New autism treatment increases IQ, makes children more normal." National TV news broadcasts picked up the story as well.

Parents, excited by the news, rushed to doctors to try to get their hands on the drug. Many of them did, despite the fact that fenfluramine was not at the time approved as an autism treatment, or as a treatment for children. But few of these parents saw the types of results claimed by the initial research study. In fact, dozens of later studies failed to detect any significant improvements in children given the drug, and several suggested that fenfluramine might cause permanent damage to brain cells. None of this information appeared in newspapers or on TV.

Even when a drug's side effects are so devastating that they do make the news, there's usually a long lag between the initial glowing reports and the later "Oops!" reports. That's what happened with Halcion, a sleeping pill introduced with a huge media splash in the late 1970s. Soon, everyone was talking about Halcion— and tens of thousands of people were taking it for symptoms ranging from minor sleeplessness to jet lag. By the time *Newsweek* asked, a decade or so later, "Is It Safe?," many of these patients had already found out, the hard way, that the answer frequently was "no." For some Halcion users, who had committed suicide or other violent acts while under the influence of the drug, it was too late.

Stories like these are all too common. Because DSM psychiatry so often fails its patients, these patients are especially vulnerable to reports of new miracle cures. The media love miracles too: they make good copy and increase ratings. But true miracle drugs are few and far between—and the odds are good that you won't learn about the real ones from TV talk shows or your morning paper.

Fad 4. The "Mental Illness Doesn't Exist" Myth

The phrase "mental illness is a myth" was coined by Thomas Szasz, a famous psychiatrist who recently told *Society* Magazine that he "took up the profession of psychiatry in part to combat the contention that abnormal behaviors are the products of abnormal brains." Szasz contends that although a handful of mental disorders are caused by biological dysfunction, most are "psychiatric fictions" that help patients escape from taking personal responsibility for their actions.

Szasz's theory, although I disagree with it, stems in part from valid criticisms of modern psychiatric practice. For instance, I can't argue with his contention, in *Mental Illness is a Myth,* that current psychiatric "diagnoses" are "driven by non-medical, that is, economic, personal, legal, political, or social considerations and incentives." I certainly agree with his charge that "anyone with an ear for language will recognize that the boundary that separates the serious vocabulary of psychiatry from the ludicrous lexicon of psychobabble, and both from playful slang, is thin and permeable to fashion." And I take no exception with him when he castigates the DSM, saying in *Society* that:

> [T]he various versions of the APA's *Diagnostic and Statistical Manual of Mental Disorders* are not classifications of mental disorders that patients have, but are rosters of officially accredited psychiatric diagnoses. This is why in psychiatry, unlike in the rest of medicine, members of consensus groups and task forces, appointed by officers of the APA, make and unmake diagnoses, the membership sometimes voting on whether a controversial diagnosis is or is not a disease.

Furthermore, I agree with Szasz that psychiatry has attempted to medicalize many variations of normal human behavior and misbehavior. As I pointed out earlier, most people labeled as "histrionic" or "avoidant" or "dependent" are perfectly normal (or at worst, slightly eccentric). And most people who blame their excesses or foolish actions on mental "illness" caused by a less-than-perfect upbringing should learn to take responsibility for their own lives.

But although Szasz is right about the fallacy of DSM "diagnoses," and about the dangers of labeling normal behavior and misbehavior as illness, he's wrong about serious brain dysfunctions being, in his words, "a neuro-mythological explanation of human wickedness." And he's dead wrong when he conjures up an imaginary line between neurological disorders, such as paresis, and "fictional" disorders such as schizophrenia.

It's ironic that Szasz, considered the leading iconoclast in the psychiatric field today, has fallen into the trap that has caught so many psychiatrists: the idea that there are "body" diseases and "mind" diseases, and that the brain has nothing to do with the mind. Szasz has gone a step further, arguing that the disorders many psychiatrists call "mental" or "functional"—that is, "all in the head"—don't exist at all. While allowing that a few patients with disorders such as neurosyphilis are legitimately crazy, Szasz suggests that most of the rest are making up their symptoms—or have been coerced by doctors and family members into believing that they are mentally ill.

Szasz's beliefs lead me to wonder how many real-life disturbed patients he has actually met. I've evaluated thousands of such patients, and, believe me, none of them was making up symptoms as a way of avoiding responsibility—nor did they make up the tumors, metabolic disorders, parasites, viruses, bacteria, brain injuries, heart defects, toxins, and medication errors that caused their symptoms. And they didn't make up the fact that their symptoms disappeared when I was able to accurately diagnose their problems and address the basic causes.

(By the way, even the patients whom DSM labels as "malingerers," and Szasz dismisses as liars, generally are suffering from brain dysfunctions. I've found, over my decades of practice, that people with normal brains rarely pretend to be crazy. Again, the brain is the organ of behavior—and aberrant behavior, even when it appears to be malingering, stems from aberrant brain functioning.)

Although I admire Szasz for being willing to take on the DSM labeling system, I'm concerned about the damage his popular books and articles are doing to patients suffering from severe brain dysfunctions. Already stigmatized, these patients don't need to be told by friends and relatives that they're perfectly fine and are simply "making up" their debilitating symptoms. They also don't need to be told that their brain dysfunction is a sign of a weak character—or that, in Szasz's words, "What we call 'sanity'—what we mean by 'not being schizophrenic'—has a great deal to do with competence, earned by struggling for excellence; with integrity, hard won by confronting conflicts; and with modesty and patience, acquired through silence and suffering." The symptoms we label as "schizophrenia"—which are clearly caused by brain disorders—are not signs of incompetence, lack of integrity, immodesty, or impatience, and blaming patients for schizophrenic symptoms is as misguided as charging that diabetes is caused by a character flaw.

As an example of how Szasz and I agree—and how we differ— let's look at the case of Rebecca Smith, discussed in Szasz's book, *The Therapeutic State*. Rebecca Smith was a homeless 61-year-old woman who spent her last days huddled in a cardboard box on a New York street. During a cold wave, Smith froze to death.

Szasz writes that Smith had spent years locked up in an insane asylum, a "treatment" that hadn't helped her a bit. He notes that she'd been given electroshock therapy and psychotropic drugs, which also didn't improve her condition. And he observes that Smith was part of the well-intentioned move, which began in the 1970s, to deinstitutionalize psychiatric patients. (Meant to "normalize" such patients, deinstitutionalization simply released into society a wave of homeless, destitute people unable to care for themselves. The results, in the form of thousands of panhandlers and street people, are now painfully clear.)

I agree with Szasz that none of the psychiatric "treatments" Smith underwent helped her, and most of them may have actively harmed her. But I don't agree with his prescription: admit "the sad truth . . . that Mrs. Smith was a person who did not take care of herself," and leave her to her own devices. "Loneliness and homelessness and the inability or unwillingness to make a life for oneself are not the symptoms of a disease," Szasz contends. But often, they are exactly that—symptoms of a brain dysfunction that, if left undiagnosed and untreated, will condemn a patient to a failed life.

What—other than "not taking care of herself"—could have caused Rebecca Smith's problems? She might have had undiagnosed Wilson's disease, a treatable condition often labeled as schizophrenia. Perhaps she had a slow-growing brain tumor, or suffered from long-term exposure to lead or other toxins, or had syphilis or porphyria. If so, leaving her to her own devices—Szasz's only prescription—would have condemned her to an entirely preventable death.

In claiming that "mental illnesses do not exist; indeed, they cannot exist, because the mind is not a body part or bodily organ," Szasz would have us dismiss millions of patients—many of whom have genetic diseases, tumors, medication-induced psychosis, infections, and other brain disorders—as incompetent, lazy, or bad. He would have us leave them to die on the streets, or in our jails. In my book, that view is as bad as the misguided psychiatric treatments Szasz rightly attacks.

Fad 5. "New Age" Psychiatry

As a preface to this section, let me stress that, unlike many doctors, I don't automatically ignore any technique labeled as "alternative medicine." I've traveled to China and learned about acupuncture, which I find highly effective as an anesthetic (although not appropriate or useful in actually treating disease). I've seen considerable scientific evidence supporting a number of orthomolecular/nutritional therapies, and I use some of them in my own practice if tests show that patients suffer from nutritional deficiencies. I believe proper breathing techniques can help alleviate symptoms of anxiety caused by hyperventilation syndrome. And one of my areas of expertise—as a medical researcher, not a practitioner!—is voodoo, which I've found to have a clearly explainable biological basis. (My fellow researchers and I found that voodoo relies on chemicals obtained from indigenous plants and fish. A chemical from the pufferfish, for instance, can induce a deathlike state, and atropine from native flowers can reverse the effect.)

In short, I've investigated a wide range of medical practices and medical philosophies, and have some credentials when it comes to evaluating the merits of alternative treatments. Furthermore, in cases where a good differential diagnosis reveals a disorder that traditional medicine can't yet treat effectively, I'd rather see patients turn to exercise, sensible eating, biofeedback, and other alternative techniques, than to harmful and potentially addictive drugs. Some alternative approaches are helpful and well-grounded scientifically, others are just plain silly, and a few are outright dangerous, but very few have as much potential for harm as psychotropic drugs do.

However, I'm seeing a dangerous trend in psychiatry, which is that "new age" techniques (frequently, those with little or no scientific basis) are *replacing*, rather than supplementing, medical treatment. One example is Ayurveda—a form of treatment based on ancient Hindu scriptures—which currently is enjoying astonishing popularity in the United States. (For instance, the highly reputed Sharp Clinic in San Diego, California, recently opened the Center for Mind Body Medicine, based on Ayurvedic medicine techniques.) Ayurveda is the hot treatment in Hollywood these days, and several books about Ayurvedic therapy have made it to the best-seller lists.

Ayurveda is based on two textual supplements to the Atharvaveda, one of the four fundamental Hindu scriptures. Jack Raso, who has studied Ayurveda extensively, notes that the Atharvaveda "features magical formulas, curses, and mystical hymns [relating] to putative botanical cures for various maladies—including conditions purportedly due to demons, ghosts, and gods." He notes, in *Nutrition Forum,* that "remedies' and 'preventives' include amulets, exorcism, invocations, and other incantations"; treatment for brain dysfunctions such as seizures, for instance, may include exorcism of evil spirits. "Magical thinking and ritualism," Raso says, ". . . are part and parcel of Ayurveda."

Some of the principles of the Ayurvedic movement are harmless and can even be beneficial. Ayurvedic practitioners stress vigorous exercise, which is vital to good health. They promote meditation, which can be very calming. And they teach breathing techniques, which, as I've noted, can be helpful in preventing anxiety. But when Ayurveda gets into "diagnosis" and "treatment," I have a problem with it.

According to Ayurvedic practitioners, there are three body types or "doshas"—vata, pitta, and kapha—and several "combination" types. A person's body type, in Ayurvedic theory, depends on the balance of five "elements"—earth, air, fire, water, and akasha ("ether")—in the body. Ayurvedic healers believe that the preponderance of these elements in each individual determines the ailments to which he or she is prone, and that disorders caused by imbalances of these forces can be treated by consuming the proper ratios of astringent, bitter, pungent, salty, sour, and sweet foods—ratios that change according to the season of the year. The "aftertaste" of foods also is believed to affect health. Enemas, bloodletting, and "therapeutic vomiting" are prescribed by some Ayurvedic practitioners—as is placing herbs up the nostrils to promote "mental clarity." In addition, patients are encouraged to use gems and crystals for their "subtle vibratory healing powers."

Ayurvedic practitioners pride themselves on their "diagnostic" methods and many scorn laboratory tests. Instead, they examine a patient's tongue, pulse, eyes, fingernails, and urine, coming up with "diagnoses" such as these: "Blackish-brown urine indicates a vata disorder; dark yellow, an imbalance with pitta." Such "diagnoses" can be made in minutes: famed Ayurvedic practitioner Deepak Chopra, in *Return of the Rishi*, tells of a Dr. Triguna, of whom a patient says, "He only has to put three fingers on your wrist, and he knows your whole medical history—past, present, and future." To a skeptical reader, the doctor's insights following this examination sound pretty obvious: "You can live a long time if you take care of this body." "You must eat more slowly." "You should walk to work in the morning." "Go to bed on time." Still, Chopra, the most noted spokesman for Ayurveda, says Triguna is a master physician, and that "even if I knew consciously that my condition was perilous, I feel that I would recover under his care. I believe in the goodness of my physician." He adds, glowingly, "I believe [Triguna] does not even see patients as bodies. They are bundles of consciousness rising to meet him."

Now, I have no complaints about what Drs. Chopra and Triguna are practicing, as long as most of it is considered as religion and not medicine. I respect my friends' and patients' religious beliefs even when I don't share them, and if someone wants to practice blood-letting, herb sniffing, or crystal gazing as part of a religious rite, it's none of my business. But *religion isn't medicine—and it isn't psychiatry*. And I *do* care if patients with treatable, curable problems forgo an accurate medical diagnosis and attempt to treat potentially lethal brain dysfunctions by balancing "hot" and "cold" foods, or performing "therapeutic vomiting"—treatments that Raso rightly describes as "nutrimedical witchcraft." I also resent the tarnishing of medicine's image by physicians who, in an effort to expand their patient base and stay trendy, promote such treatments in the absence of any research showing that they work. This is, purely and simply, hucksterism.

Why Is Pop Psychiatry so Popular?

Why do so many people suffering from psychiatric disorders turn to mysticism, primal scream therapy, "codependency" therapy, repressed memory therapy, and other nonmedical treatments? And why do they rush to their doctors to demand each new fad drug the media promotes? Not because they're foolish, but because the only other approach they know of—psychiatry—has abandoned them. If DSM psychiatry assigns you a meaningless label and tells you that your only treatment options are drugs or psychotherapy, and neither one cures your problems, then you'll look elsewhere—and the more desperate you become, the more willingly you'll consider even far-out therapies. Pop psychiatry wouldn't be successful if it didn't fill a huge vacuum created by traditional psychiatry.

In any field of medicine, the number of patients seeking far-out cures and miracle drugs is a good index of the field's failure to cure disease. Often, this failure is unavoidable; for instance, despite our best efforts, we can't yet cure patients with AIDS or end-stage lung cancer. But in the case of DSM psychiatry, the failure to help patients is doubly tragic because—as we've seen—most of these patients could be diagnosed, and many of them could be cured.

There's another reason why "new age" therapies such as Ayurveda are popular: psychoanalytically oriented psychiatrists, who ruled the field until recently, have taught patients to accept the idea that psychiatric treatment is a mystical, quasi-religious experience. (Writer Martin Gross goes so far as to call psychoanalytic psychiatry "religion under the cloak of science.") Like priests, psychoanalytically oriented psychiatrists have always cultivated the idea that they deal in an intangible: for priests, it's the "spirit"; for psychiatrists, it's the "psyche." And like religion, psychiatry has expected its followers to take its claims on faith, rather than expecting proof. There has been less scientific investigation of psychiatric practices than of any other field of medicine. To a great degree, psychiatry has paved the way for "medical" treatments based on myth and mysticism rather than on provable facts, documented research, and scientific diagnostic methods.

How can psychiatry stop the spread of silly pop psychiatry and pop psychology offshoots, and reverse the field's devolutionary spiral into quackery and New Age supernaturalism? By diagnosing and treating patients' underlying disorders, rather than merely giving them DSM labels and sending them away dissatisfied. By asserting itself as a science, based on the idea that *the brain is the organ of behavior*. And by abandoning the pretense that psychiatry deals in the unknowable and intangible realm of the psyche and, instead, treating brain dysfunction as a medical, not a spiritual, problem.

CHAPTER 7

How to Protect Yourself, and Those You Love, from Misdiagnosis

Health and intellect are the two blessings of life.

Menander, circa 300 B.C.

So far, I've looked at what psychiatry needs to do in order to grow beyond its stagnant DSM mentality. But change needs to come not just from within the profession, but from the patients who use psychiatric services. By taking more responsibility for their own health, and by demanding better care from their physicians—and particularly their psychiatrists—health care consumers can play a vital role in the next psychiatric revolution.

To find out how, let's look at a typical psychiatric patient.

Bob is an average all-American guy. He doesn't exercise, he drinks five cups of coffee in the morning and three beers each night, he smokes half a pack of cigarettes a day, and he lives on hamburgers and french fries, but all in all, he feels pretty good.

Then, suddenly, Bob has an anxiety attack. His heart pounds wildly, he grows dizzy, and he breaks out in a cold sweat. His legs feel like rubber. His hands shake, and he feels as though he's going to faint. It's over after a few minutes—but the next week he has another attack, and then another. Soon the attacks are occurring three or four times a day.

Bob gets scared. He visits an HMO physician listed in a booklet provided by his insurance company. The physician, after a

162

cursory physical that reveals nothing, suggests that Bob is suffering from job-related stress. He's referred to another HMO-approved doctor at a local for-profit psychiatric facility where, after another cursory examination, he gets a DSM "diagnosis" of anxiety disorder, a prescription for benzodiazepines, and a referral to a psychotherapist. When the medications don't help, Bob's psychiatrist increases the dosage. Meanwhile, his therapist suggests that his problems may stem from "codependency," and recommends extensive counseling for him and his entire family.

What's wrong with this picture? In my opinion, just about everything. Yet it's typical of the experiences of patients with brain dysfunctions.

Bob and his doctors, collectively, have virtually guaranteed that he'll get worse instead of better. And although it's tempting (and correct) to lay much of the blame on Bob's general practitioner and his psychiatrist, Bob has to share in the guilt. From abdicating responsibility for his own health, to "bargain shopping" for health care, to unquestioningly accepting a DSM label, poor treatment, and dangerous medications, Bob has been an accomplice in his own deficient health care.

What can you do to avoid the trap Bob fell into?

Let's start with the obvious: *Your health is your most priceless possession.* There is nothing—I repeat, *nothing*—more important than taking care of your health. This is particularly true of your brain's health, because although a person can lead a fulfilling life with a bad kidney or an arthritic knee, brain dysfunction by its nature takes away the very substance of an individual. There is *nothing* more important than protecting your brain's integrity while you're well and receiving good care when you're not.

So protect the health of your body and brain to the greatest extent possible. And, if you do suffer a brain disorder, think like a consumer—not like a patient. Seek out the best opinion/diagnosis you can find, even if that means disagreeing with your insurers, your physicians, or your employer about what level of medical care is "good enough." As Charles Inlander, president of the People's

Medical Society, has said, "Medical mistakes have occurred and continue to occur because we have been lax customers." Think of the work that goes into buying a good car, purchasing furniture, or maintaining a yard or a home. Isn't your health—particularly your mental health—more important than any of these?

There are some specific steps a smart consumer of psychiatric services can take to minimize the need for medical care, maximize the quality of care received, and avoid falling into the DSM trap. In cases where patients are too impaired to take charge of their own care, their families can follow these steps.

Avoid Self-Inflicted Brain Disorders

The English philosopher Herbert Spencer once said, "The preservation of health is a duty." It's also just plain smart, because fixing a damaged body is a lot harder than keeping it in shape in the first place. Yet most of us spend fortunes maintaining our cars and homes, while subjecting our bodies to too much bad food, too little sleep, too little exercise, and too much alcohol.

I'm not implying that all (or even most) cases of brain dysfunction stem from bad health habits. The majority result from a bad roll of the genetic dice, or an unavoidable disease or injury. But quite a few others result, partially or wholly, from poor health practices. Many DSM labels are simply cover-ups for poor health practices that have taken their toll on brain function.

Take our friend Bob. While he may be suffering from some unavoidable disorder, it's equally likely that his panic attacks originally stemmed from caffeinism (from his excessive coffee drinking), or hyperinsulinism (from his bad diet and overconsumption of alcohol). His anxiety and dizziness may be symptoms of inner-ear problems, which can be brought on by cardiovascular disease—something Bob's smoking and bad diet could have caused. His weight and his sedentary lifestyle aren't doing his brain any good, either.

Virtually any vice that's bad for the body is bad for the brain. Excessive alcohol consumption destroys brain cells and reduces the liver's ability to remove toxins that can alter brain function. Smoking increases the risk of stroke, decreases blood flow to the brain, and increases levels of carbon monoxide and other toxins. Overeating congests arteries with cholesterol (again, decreasing blood flow to the brain). A bad diet deprives the brain of nutrients—the building blocks of brain chemicals—and can "starve" the brain by reducing levels of the glucose it uses for fuel. Lack of exercise reduces oxygen flow to the brain, and lowers levels of natural "feel-good" chemicals called endorphins. Poor sleeping habits change circadian rhythms—the body's natural patterns of eating, sleeping, waking, and energy—and can have dramatic effects on brain chemicals. Promiscuous sex is a risk factor for syphilis and other venereal diseases that can affect the brain.

You don't have to live like a monk, of course. An occasional ice cream sundae or a day off from exercising is good for you (I confess that I indulge in a pipe). You don't need to be a tireless health fanatic, but the healthier your lifestyle is, the less your risk of brain dysfunction. Be health-conscious at your job and your hobbies as well. If you're going to play football or ride a bike, wear a helmet. If you're working with toxic chemicals, limit your exposure. Don't get carried away worrying about every little health risk, but do try to avoid the big ones. The best way to stay out of the DSM trap is to avoid developing a brain dysfunction in the first place.

Don't Mismedicate or Overmedicate Yourself

One of the biggest risks to your mental health (and your health in general) is the misuse or overuse of prescription and nonprescription medications. A recent extensive study determined that *one-fourth* of people over age 65 in the United States are taking drugs that are inappropriate and potentially dangerous. And millions of

Americans, young and old, are taking multiple drugs that can interact—often dangerously—with each other in unexpected ways. This overmedication has serious consequences: millions of adults suffer from adverse drug reactions each year, and tens of thousands of them die.

Many of the prescription and over-the-counter (OTC) drugs Americans take can affect brain function. Diet pills, in addition to possibly increasing the risk of cardiac arrest, can cause anxiety and other "mental" symptoms. Some antifungal drugs can cause severe psychiatric disturbance in people with porphyria. Certain ulcer drugs are poorly metabolized by older patients and can cause thought impairment or even outright dementia. Blood pressure medications can cause severe mood changes, sexual problems, and distorted thinking. Chronic aspirin use can lead to anemia, which can cause lethargy, sadness, and hopelessness. Nonsteroidal anti-inflammatory drugs (NSAIDS) can impair blood flow to the kidneys in some individuals, increasing the risk of personality changes, confusion, and memory loss. And antihistamines, sleeping medications, and antacids can contribute to nervous system dysfunction either directly (by affecting brain cells) or indirectly (by disrupting other bodily processes critical to brain function). Reactions to medications are so common, in fact, that I devoted nearly one-third of my first book, *Psychiatric Signs and Symptoms Due to Medical Problems,* to describing drug reactions that can result in behavioral abnormalities.

Many prescription drugs, of course, serve a useful or even a vital purpose. But even necessary medications need to be monitored carefully and should be adjusted if any unusual behavioral symptoms occur. Drug monitoring is particularly important for older patients, who have slower metabolism rates and are thus more vulnerable to drug side effects.

A typical case of drug-related "mental" problems, which I witnessed in my own practice, involved Gladys, a 90-year-old woman who was a favorite at her residential facility because of her sweet disposition and quick sense of humor. Gladys was dubbed the "welcome wagon lady" by staffers, because she made the rounds every day, putting on her hat and pearls and checking up on every resident. If she found someone who was feeling despondent, Gladys—who never took "no" for an answer—would drag the reluctant sulker off to a painting class, sing-a-long, or other facility activity. She even checked up on the staff members, who quickly learned to "put on a happy face" when she was around.

The staff at Gladys's facility was surprised and alarmed when she didn't make her rounds one day. Shortly afterward, when Gladys became disoriented and started having hallucinations, her physician admitted her to a local hospital. Staff members brought her personal medications to the hospital, including the eyedrops she was using to treat her glaucoma. However, the eyedrops ran out during her first week in the hospital. Remarkably, as soon as she stopped using the drops, Glayds's behavior returned to normal. By the time I was asked to evaluate her, a few days later, she was bright and active, was capable of caring for herself again, and showed no signs of central nervous system dysfunction. Pretty soon, she was visiting the other patients on her floor—and asking her doctors how they were doing.

The cause of Gladys's "mental" illness proved, indeed, to be her eyedrops. Pilocarpine (the drug in Gladys's eyedrops) and similar medications work by mimicking the effects of acetylcholine, one of the brain's messenger chemicals. The drugs reduce pupil size and lower fluid pressure within the eye, but they also can cause acute brain dysfunction. (The lesson here, again, is that there is no "magic bullet"; every drug causes unwanted as well as desired effects, and this is particularly true of drugs that enhance or block the effects of brain chemicals.) Although glaucoma medications are a valuable treatment, people who use them should be aware of this potential problem, and notify their doctors if they experience any unusual symptoms.

In *The Safe Medicine Book,* Kathryn Watterson tells a similar story about an 81-year-old woman who suddenly underwent a drastic personality change. "This woman, who had always been a happy and emotionally generous person, was calling her niece a slut and a whore, [and] cursing her deceased husband," Watterson says. Admitted to a hospital, she roamed the halls, yelling obscenities and hallucinating. The cause of her terrible symptoms? A new heart medication prescribed by her physician. The medicine was stopped, and Watterson reports that "within 48 hours she was normal again." In the same book, Watterson tells of an attorney whose blood pressure medication, Captopril (which alters levels of several brain chemicals), caused such severe despondency that within 20 minutes of getting up each morning "he would crawl back into bed, curl up in a fetal position, and tell [his wife] he was just waiting to die." The drug was stopped, and the man's symptoms disappeared within four days.

Even physicians are often surprised at the severity of "mental" symptoms that can be brought on by seemingly innocuous prescription or OTC medications. Psychiatrist Abraham Twerski, for instance, tells the story of a brief "depressive" episode that occurred when he began taking a new decongestant for his hay fever. "I began to notice I was losing interest in things and had difficulty concentrating," Twerski wrote, in *Who Says You're Neurotic?* "Shortly thereafter I lost my appetite, and all food seemed to taste like cardboard. . . . Then I began awakening at 2:00 A.M., feeling agitated, trapped and doomed to be this way forever." Just about the time he decided to seek psychiatric help, he suddenly realized that his dramatic mood changes coincided with his medication change. He stopped using the medication, and his hay fever returned—but, more importantly, his terrible depression cleared up within days.

Taking drugs—any drugs—can be risky. Use them if you need them, but only if you really *do* need them. And if you experience any unusual symptoms, including "mental" symptoms, check with a doctor immediately and ask whether the drug may be contributing to your problems. Remember, even prescription drugs used for legitimate purposes can cause severe and dangerous side effects. Every person is different, and every person reacts differently to a drug.

Feeling Blue or Anxious or Tired? Play Detective

If you do develop mild anxiety, moodiness, or "blahs," try doing a little detective work yourself before heading to a physician (and particularly a psychiatrist). Many minor problems that psychiatrists mislabel as DSM disorders—particularly the self-inflicted health problems I discussed above—can be self-diagnosed fairly readily. (You'll find the 24-hour-day profile, on pages 170–171, helpful in this endeavor.)

Start by keeping track of your activities for several weeks—including workdays and weekends. Then answer the following questions.

Is there anything unusual about your eating or sleeping patterns?

Are your symptoms correlated with specific activities?

Do your symptoms vary according to what you eat or drink?

Do your symptoms occur at work but not at home, or vice versa?

Do your symptoms occur when you're active, or when you're relaxing?

Do your symptoms occur when you've had too much to drink, or too little sleep?

Are your symptoms associated with the use of solvents, insecticides, or other toxic chemicals?

Are your symptoms worse outdoors or indoors?

Does your daily routine suggest a chronically unhealthy lifestyle?

Are you burning the candle at both ends, or grabbing too many junk-food meals on the run?

Do you spend all day in an office with no windows?

Do you work long hours and spend too little time enjoying yourself or exercising?

Do you spend too many hours eating potato chips in front of the TV?

The 24-Hour-Day

Answers to these questions can help you pinpoint the causes of your own minor emotional or behavioral problems, or can offer valuable clues to an alert physician. If you're planning to visit a psychiatrist or other physician because you're experiencing sadness, memory problems, anxiety, or other emotional or behavioral problems, go through this list and make a note of any "red flags" you spot. Be sure to report this information to your doctor—even if he or she doesn't ask.

What time do you go to bed?

Are you sleepy at that time, or is this just a routine?

Do you have any rituals before going to bed?

Do you sleep on a regular bed or a waterbed? Alone or with a partner?

How long does it take you to fall asleep? Do you use sleeping medication?

If you have trouble falling asleep, how long does it take you to fall asleep?

Are you a deep sleeper or a light sleeper? Are you easily awakened, or do you need to be shaken to be awakened?

Are you a restless sleeper? When you wake up, are your bedclothes a mess?

Do you clench or grind your teeth, snore, sleepwalk, get up to go to the bathroom, or drink water during the night?

Do you get up to eat?

Are you awakened by a partner's snoring or restless sleep?

Do you sleep on your back, your side, or your stomach? Do you sleep with your arm under your head? How many pillows do you use?

Is your jaw tense when you wake up?

Do you wet or soil the bed?

Do you sleep with the windows open or closed?

If you speak several languages, which one do you dream in? Is it your native language, or one you mastered later?

What time do you wake up in the morning?

(Continued)

(Continued)

Do you awaken refreshed, or are you still tired?

Do you eat breakfast? If so, what?

Do you drink coffee with breakfast? If so, how much?

Do you feel better or worse after breakfast?

Do you go to the office after breakfast, or work at home?

Do you have plenty of energy to do your morning tasks?

Do you drink coffee during the morning? If so, how much?

Do you snack during the morning? If so, what do you snack on?

Do you nap in the morning? If so, how long are your naps, and how do you feel when you awaken?

What work do you do? Do you work around chemicals, fumes, or potentially toxic materials?

Do you eat lunch? If so, when? What do you eat?

How do you feel before lunch? After lunch?

Do you have sufficient energy during the afternoon to do your work? Do you have more energy in the afternoon or in the morning?

Do you drink coffee in the afternoon? If so, how much?

Do you snack in the afternoon? If so, what do you eat?

Do you nap in the afternoon? If so, how long are your naps, and how do you feel when you awaken?

What do you do after work (exercise, recreation, etc.)?

What time do you have dinner? What do you have? Do you have drinks before, during, or after dinner? If so, what type and how many? Do you have coffee? If so, how much?

What do you do after dinner (hobbies, exercise, etc.)?

Do you snack after dinner?

Do you use a gas heater at night?

What medications, vitamins, or over-the-counter drugs do you take?

Whom do you see during the day (family members, boyfriends or girlfriends, etc.)? What activities do you and your friends participate in?

At what times during the day do your symptoms worsen? At what time do they bother you the least?

Pay particular attention, when examining your activities during the day and night, to situations that either bring on or alleviate your symptoms. For instance, if your symptoms occur when you're home but not at work, check your gas heater or stove. Many people—particularly elderly people living in substandard housing—suffer from low-grade carbon monoxide poisoning, which reduces the supply of oxygen to the brain and causes a wide range of "mental" symptoms such as chronic fatigue, sadness, despair, hopelessness, and sleepiness. Even very minor carbon monoxide poisoning can cause grogginess and memory loss.

You may find that the explanation for your symptoms is even more simple. Maybe your anxiety started when you switched from decaf to regular coffee. Maybe your dizzy spells always occur after skipping lunch and eating sugary snacks. Maybe your headaches and fatigue stem from the poor air circulation in a new "energy-efficient" home. Maybe you just need a vacation. If you pinpoint a possible culprit, eliminate it if you can, and see if your symptoms go away.

You may also find, if your symptoms are mild, that what I call the "tincture of time" will eliminate them. In other words, many problems, given some time, clear up by themselves. Studies have shown, in fact, that up to two-thirds of all patients seeking psychotherapy get over their problems while still waiting for appointments. (Interestingly, about the same number of patients are cured by psychotherapists!) Voltaire's famous saying, "The art of medicine consists of amusing the patient while nature cures the disease," is particularly apt as it relates to minor behavioral and emotional symptoms. Such recoveries aren't surprising, because the body is designed to be self-healing. It's good at excreting toxins, fighting off viral infections, and regaining balance after an environmental insult.

The advice above applies only to minor problems. If you are experiencing *any* serious symptoms, or have experienced symptoms for some time, or realize that your symptoms are progressively worsening, it's important to seek medical advice immediately. But here again, the 24-hour-day profile can be invaluable. Go through the list, and write down everything unusual about your eating, sleeping, and activity patterns, no matter how minor. Tell your doctor about your findings—even if he or she doesn't ask. Also provide your physician with information about any hobbies, trips to foreign countries, use of prescription and over-the-counter medications, job changes, or other life changes, large or small, that might have a bearing on your problems. The more details you give your doctor, the less likely it is that you will be given an inadequate diagnosis or a DSM label.

Consider a Psychiatrist as a Last Resort

As I've said earlier, most psychiatrists practice DSM medicine, and DSM labels are cover-ups—not diagnoses—for real medical disorders. Therefore, your best bet in seeking an accurate diagnosis is to start with a *non*psychiatric physician.

In most cases, your first visit (but *not* your only visit) should be to your general practitioner (GP). If you're suffering from a fairly common ailment, a GP might be able to solve your problem readily. Bear in mind, however, that most general practitioners don't have the time or the specialized office equipment necessary to diagnose complex or unusual problems. Furthermore, more and more GPs are being programmed by the American Psychiatric Association to label patients as "depressed" and to refer them immediately to psychiatrists (or prescribe antidepressants themselves).

If your general practitioner is unable to uncover the source of your symptoms (which often will be the case), then ask for a referral to an appropriate specialist—which, in most cases, *won't* be a psychiatrist. If your symptoms include heart palpitations and anxiety, for instance, see a cardiologist. If you're experiencing both despondency and digestive upsets, see an internal medicine specialist. If you suffer from dizziness, see a neurologist or an ear/nose/throat doctor (who is trained to recognize disorders of the vestibular system inside the ear). If you're age 70 or older, a "geriatrician"—a doctor who specializes in treating older patients—may be the best choice. And if all of your symptoms appear to be "in your mind," make an appointment with a neurologist rather than a psychiatrist. In general, it's a good idea to investigate all other likely medical approaches before making an appointment with a psychiatrist.

Be sure, when you see a nonpsychiatric specialist, that he or she conducts a thorough exam and investigates all of your complaints instead of simply passing you on to a psychiatrist. Too often, nonpsychiatric physicians consider the presence of any "mental" symptom grounds for a psychiatric referral—even when other symptoms abound. Thus, as David Gross and colleagues note, in *Medical Mimics of Psychiatric Disorders,* "The patient with chronic abdominal pain, DSM criteria for major depression, and a non-specific physical examination and laboratory screening becomes a psychiatric patient for want of a better diagnosis." Furthermore, some nonpsychiatric physicians make psychiatric referrals prematurely because they are uncomfortable around patients with brain dysfunction. "Because of the presence of abnormal and often bizarre mental states," Gross and his coauthors say, "psychiatric patients may instill a generalized uneasiness in consultants." Try to find an empathetic doctor who understands that "mental" symptoms are medical symptoms, and who is willing to evaluate you as a medical patient—not as a psychiatric patient.

And watch out for "DSM syndrome" even in your general practitioner's office—because in 1995, the American Psychiatric Association, in its continuing effort to expand DSM's role, created a separate edition of DSM aimed specifically at nonpsychiatric physicians (particularly, general practitioners). The DSM-IV for Primary Care (DSM-IV-PC), according to an article in *Physicians Financial News,* "will present algorithms [a fancy term for cookbook lists] for determining the presence of a psychiatric disorder, beginning with the types of symptoms most commonly seen in primary-care practices, such as depressed mood, anxiety, *unexplained general medical conditions,* impaired memory and substance abuse [emphasis added]." In other words, the general practitioner, like the psychiatrist, will now have an excuse to explain away "unexplained"—in other words, undiagnosed—medical conditions by dismissing them as symptoms of "mental" disorders.

This is particularly likely to happen to patients experiencing any of the symptoms commonly labeled as "depression." Massive promotion of antidepressants by drug companies, combined with DSM's legitimization of "depression" as a disease in and of itself, have led general practitioners to write millions of prescriptions for antidepressant drugs—and to shortcut their investigations into the real causes of their patients' symptoms. One 1993 study found that more than half of the doctors the researchers surveyed wrote prescriptions for "depression" after visiting with a patient *for less than three minutes.*

A story told by Siegfried Kra, a physician and professor of medicine at Yale, illustrates just how dangerous such diagnostic shortcuts can be. In *Aging Myths,* Kra tells of Bill, a 54-year-old insurance salesman who became impotent. In addition, Bill started suffering from despondency and terrible fatigue, and his wife noticed that he was having memory problems. At Bill's initial checkup, his doctor advised him to take a vacation; he did, but his symptoms persisted. So he returned to his doctor, who labeled him as suffering from depression caused by a "midlife crisis," and prescribed antidepressants. The drugs didn't help Bill at all. Kra notes that a neighbor, admiring Bill's tan, remarked, "I don't know what's bothering Bill. He looks so healthy, yet he feels so lousy."

That healthy-looking tan, it turned out, wasn't healthy at all. A second, more savvy doctor, whose curiosity was piqued by Bill's dark coloring, examined him closely and found "dirty" looking areas around his genitals and brown spots inside his mouth. As Kra tells it, "The combination of exhaustion, feebleness, the brown coloration of the skin, and the brown spots in the mouth were the clues that the doctor needed to make the diagnosis of adrenocortical insufficiency, or failure of the adrenal glands." His disorder—called Addison's disease—was easy to treat. Within a short time, Kra reports, Bill's impotence, depression, fatigue, and memory loss vanished.

Five Questions to Answer before Seeing a Psychiatrist

1. Have you had a thorough and satisfactory examination by a family practitioner and/or appropriate medical specialist before considering a psychiatrist?

2. Have you obtained a second (or third, or fourth) opinion, and are you prepared to be assertive in questioning a psychiatrist's diagnosis?

3. Are you practicing poor health habits (drinking too much coffee, smoking cigarettes) or poor sleep habits that may be responsible for your not feeling like yourself?

4. Are your feelings or behavior patterns normal reactions to life events (for example, pressure at work, loss of a loved one, etc.)?

5. What medications, vitamins, or over-the-counter drugs are you currently taking?

Cases like Bill's aren't rare, and some patients are particularly at risk. Among them are people over 60, who are often misdiagnosed as having "depression" or "dementia," and children, who are being labeled as "hyperactive" by general practitioners at an alarming rate (more on both of these high-risk groups later). And be especially wary of DSM syndrome if you're a woman: a number of studies show that doctors dismiss women's complaints as psychosomatic far more often than they do men's complaints. One survey, in which doctors received lists of male and female patients' symptoms and were asked to suggest diagnoses, found that the female patients' symptoms were more likely to be labeled as "all in their heads"—even when the women's symptoms were exactly the same as the men's.

So even when you visit a nonpsychiatric physician, you may be "DSMed"—but at least your odds of getting an accurate differential diagnosis are better. A cardiologist isn't likely to write off your heart palpitations as functional without at least conducting studies, and an internal medicine physician isn't likely to call your intestinal problems psychogenic without checking to see whether you have an inflammatory bowel disease.

Five Questions You Should Ask
If You *Do* Go to a Psychiatrist

1. Does your psychiatrist believe that DSM labels, such as "hyperactivity" and "depression," are the same as real medical diagnoses, and does he or she base treatments on such labels?
2. Will your visit include an extensive medical history evaluation and physical examination, as well as appropriate laboratory tests?
3. If your tests and examination reveal a biological disorder, will the drug your psychiatrist prescribes correct the problem or simply mask its symptoms?
4. Is your psychiatrist recommending psychotherapy for your condition, and, if so, is the psychotherapy being prescribed *in addition to* medical diagnosis and treatment, or *instead of* medical diagnosis and treatment?
5. How would your psychiatrist compare the risks and benefits of any drugs he or she recommends?

That being the case, the psychiatrist should almost always be a last, not a first, resort. If other specialists fail to diagnose the cause of your problems, however, you may eventually need to consult a psychiatrist. If that happens, the advice that follows may help you select a good doctor—and get the right kind of care once you find one.

Bargain-Basement Medical Care Is Worth What You Pay for It

You've heard that Doctor Smith is an excellent psychiatrist who takes pains to properly diagnose and treat patients—but your company's health plan only covers visits to Dr. Jones. So you make an appointment with Dr. Jones, figuring that your company plan's doctors should be as good as any in private practice.

Bad decision.

You might have a difficult time making the *right* decision in these circumstances, because it's getting harder and harder to find a private psychiatrist. Private practice physicians in general are an endangered species, increasingly being shoved aside by doctors working for health maintenance organizations (HMOs) and preferred provider organizations (PPOs). "Eight years ago," Sacramento Medical Society executive director William Sandberg told *American Medical News* recently, "70 percent of physicians were in solo practice—today it's only 30 percent." And if you choose to visit a doctor in private practice, your company's insurance program will most likely pay far less (or even none) of your costs.

So why should you pay good out-of-pocket money for a private practice psychiatrist? Because, for the private psychiatrist, the patient's health is the bottom line. But the HMO/PPO doctor has divided loyalties: to the patient, who deserves good care, and to the organization, which demands that corners be cut at every opportunity. The HMO/PPO doctor is forced to make compromises, and, in doing so, to put patients at risk. The HMO or PPO limits the number of tests a doctor can order, the number of minutes patients' exams should last, and the number of days physicians can keep patients in the hospital. These magic formulas too often are thought up not by physicians, but by nonmedical business managers who are more concerned with the bottom line than with any individual patient. Furthermore, HMOs and PPOs encourage "cookie cutter" medicine by attempting to standardize care, neglecting the fact that human beings don't come off an assembly line.

I'm not saying that there's no place for HMOs and PPOs. When it comes to treating sprained ankles or chicken pox, an HMO/PPO doctor can provide adequate care. But if you have a serious illness—particularly one that is subtle and difficult to diagnose, as many forms of brain dysfunction are—"managed care" can be risky. There's no advantage in saving a few hundred dollars up front if you're risking nondiagnosis or incomplete diagnosis, and improper or even dangerous treatments. This is especially true of psychiatry, where cutting corners too often means assigning a DSM label and handing out a prescription in the absence of even a minimal evaluation.

By the way, doctors who insist on remaining in private practice rather than succumbing to the pressure to join HMOs and PPOs don't do so out of greed. (In fact, most doctors who remain in private practice are severely punished financially by insurers, who steer most of their patients to other doctors.) For the overwhelming majority of physicians who retain their independence, the deciding factor is not money but quality of patient care. The private practice physicians I know have avoided HMOs and PPOs because they refuse to go along with what a recent article in the *Journal of the American Medical Association* described as a system that relies on "exclusion of sicker patients, rationing by inconvenience, burdensome micromanagement of clinical decisions, or denial of beneficial but expensive care to some patients, either by micromanagement or by perverse incentives for providers."

HMOs and PPOs are the latest development in a trend that is changing medicine from a noble calling into a commodity market. The trend started several decades ago, when large numbers of nonprofit hospitals, often charitable institutions run by religious orders, were bought by for-profit hospital chains. Admittedly, such buyouts saved many a hospital from going under financially, but they also changed the focus of hospitals. (A hospital run by a nun has a vastly different "institutional attitude" than one run by a CEO with a major in business administration!) Far too often, unfortunately, the focus is now on profits rather than on offering patients the best possible treatment.

Beware the For-Profit Psychiatric Hospital Chains

The trend toward commercialization of medical care has affected psychiatry as well: chains of for-profit psychiatric facilities have sprung up around the country, quickly becoming a big business.

Unfortunately, the business is based, far too often, on profit rather than patients' health.

If that sounds cynical, consider the evidence. In 1971, before most insurance plans covered psychiatric hospital stays, only 6,500 children and teenagers were hospitalized in private psychiatric facilities in the United States. Now that such insurance coverage is common, up to a quarter of a million children are admitted to psychiatric hospitals annually. By 1989, according to a Blue Cross representative, more than 30 percent of all inpatient days for Blue Cross patients were for admissions to psychiatric hospitals—and psychiatric hospitals are running huge marketing campaigns to increase these figures. "Worst of all," the Blue Cross official told a writer for *The Doctor's People,* "there's very little evidence that this upsurge in inpatient treatment is working."

There is growing evidence, on the other hand, of a system that has been corrupted in the pursuit of higher profits. In 1992, the U.S. House of Representatives Select Committee on Children, Youth, and Families reported that its investigations had uncovered instances of for-profit psychiatric hospitals paying bonuses to employees for "recruiting" patients; keeping patients against their will until insurance payments ran out; and even paying kickbacks to school guidance counselors for referring students as patients. Mike Moncrief, chairman of the Texas Senate Interim Committee on Health and Human Services, investigated psychiatric hospitals in his area and testified that "time and time again . . . witnesses gave accounts of how they were cured miraculously on the day their insurance benefits ran out. . . . Others related horrifying experiences of having voluntarily sought treatment for such conditions as an eating disorder or chronic back pain and then finding themselves being held against their will. Still others told of having their diagnosis falsified by hospital personnel so it would match their insurance benefits."

As Moncrief's testimony indicates, many psychiatric hospitals have learned how to play the DSM game for financial gain. To psychiatric hospitals, DSM labels are to a large degree a means of sorting out the patients they want from the patients they don't want. "The ambiguities involved in using (or ignoring) DSM diagnostic criteria allow agencies discretion and a rationale for accepting, rejecting, or referring an applicant for service," Stuart Kirk and Herb Kutchins say, in *The Selling of DSM*. "A clinic offering a special program for people with 'mood disorders' may need operationally to liberalize their interpretation of the criteria when in need of clients and narrow it when their caseloads are full." Thus, if you go to the hospital on Friday, when there are empty beds, you may be labeled as "mood disordered;" if you go the next Tuesday, when the beds are filled, you may be told that you have a less serious problem not requiring hospitalization. As Kirk and Kutchins note, the DSM system "is easily manipulated by staff to control client flow into and out of facilities."

In the same manner, reimbursement for psychiatric hospital treatment is often manipulated by the use of DSM labels. In 1991, law enforcement agencies in several states charged private psychiatric hospitals with routinely misdiagnosing (or rather, "mislabeling") patients in order to increase insurance reimbursement.

My own experiences with private, for-profit psychiatric hospitals have done little to reassure me that patients' well-being is at the top of their list of goals. For instance, I was called to consult recently on a case involving an elderly man who was admitted to a psychiatric facility after he became "psychotic" while recuperating from surgery for lung cancer. The facility wanted me to give him a DSM label; instead, I cured him. (It wasn't difficult to determine that his sudden symptoms stemmed from biochemical imbalances caused by one of the medications he was given following his surgery.) If you think the facility was pleased by this development, guess again; they seemed quite put out by the situation, and I haven't had a referral from them since.

So be wary of "corporate medicine." Pick a doctor with your interests, not an HMO board's, at heart. And don't select a for-profit psychiatric facility solely on the basis of its touching TV ads, because the advertisements for psychiatric hospitals bear little relationship to reality.

How *do* you find a good psychiatrist? One way is to ask your family doctor to whom he or she would send friends or relatives. Another good option is to network, through support groups or computer contacts, with individuals experiencing similar problems. Don't be swayed, however, by reports that a physician is "nice." Nice is good in a physician, but smart is better. (All physicians have known charming doctors whose patients, influenced by a lovely bedside manner, were blind to the atrocious care they received.) Instead, if you talk to people who have been to a particular psychiatrist, ask (if you can do so politely) how much time the doctor spent with them, how many questions (and what types of questions) he or she asked, how carefully he or she listened to the patient, and whether the patient got a DSM label or a real diagnosis.

Physician Jay Goldstein, author of *Could Your Doctor Be Wrong?*, offers the following suggestions for patients seeking good doctors: "Beware of the doctor who dismisses everything out of hand and who doesn't want to get into the unusual symptoms you have. . . . [B]eware of any doctor who says, in whatever terms, 'It's all in your head!' . . . Look for a physician who will listen carefully and be able to apply a broad base of knowledge to your problem to come up with a sound diagnosis and appropriate treatment."

"Above all," Goldstein says, "don't settle for second-best medicine. If you have a problem, you deserve to have it considered for what it is. If your doctor tries to make your problem fit a cookbook diagnosis, he's doing you a disservice."

Once you find a good doctor—which may take some effort—be as patient as he or she is. Remember that *an accurate diagnosis often takes time,* and there are no shortcuts.

I vividly remember Lisa, a young patient of mine, who came to me after coming unglued while undergoing repressed memory therapy during her senior year in college. Although I suspected that many of Lisa's problems were caused by her therapist, I also found that she had subtle symptoms of brain dysfunction—symptoms that had probably troubled her enough to make her want therapy in the first place. To pinpoint the causes of her problems, I told Lisa, we'd need to run several biochemical studies.

But Lisa had come to me expecting an instant diagnosis and a prescription. She'd read Peter Kramer's *Listening to Prozac,* and she demanded to know why I hadn't heard that "there's a drug for what I've got." She became frustrated at my lengthy diagnostic procedures, and found a doctor willing to give her a DSM label and write her a prescription for Prozac. Lisa's underlying problems—which I'd already begun narrowing down, thanks to abnormal lab results—remained untreated. Worse yet, the Prozac, far from alleviating Lisa's existing problems, led to bizarre personality changes: the once well-mannered and meek young lady turned into a Jezebel who embarrassed her father's business associates and caused no end of grief to her parents. Her mother called, about a year after she'd started on Prozac, to say she'd run off with a 70-year-old friend of the family.

I know it's hard to be patient when you're suffering, but when it comes to medical care, you're better off waiting a few weeks for a diagnosis and treatment than getting a "quick fix" like Lisa's. So give your physician time. The more time he or she takes, the more likely you are to be diagnosed and treated—and the less likely you are to add to your existing problems.

Be Sure You're Seeing a Medical Doctor

Many mental health functions are now performed by nonpsychiatrists: social workers, counselors, and psychologists. All of these professionals offer valid services, but none of them is qualified to diagnose brain dysfunction—even though most of them are experts in the art of DSM labeling.

This caveat also applies to professionals in the relatively new field of neuropsychology. The batteries of tests that neuropsychologists perform can offer valuable information for researchers and can be useful to psychiatrists in some cases as an *adjunct* to medical tests, but they are not medical tests in and of themselves. Unfortunately, neuropsychologists are often consulted by both neurologists and psychiatrists seeking to determine the organicity of an ailment— that is, whether a patient has a "real" brain disorder. In fact, many physicians, unaware of the limitations of psychological testing, rely so heavily on such tests that a psychologist's report reading "No evidence of organicity" becomes a green light for treating a patient's problem as purely psychological, with no further questions asked. Yet evaluations of neuropsychological testing techniques prove that their ability to detect organic disorders often is no better than random. For instance, studies by David Faust and his associates found that professional neuropsychologists, evaluating the results of standard intellectual tests, could not detect when study subjects were faking brain dysfunction (even though these adolescent subjects had been given no instructions by the researchers other than to "be convincing").

Most of the psychological tests used today have been developed by nonmedical mental health professionals who have little background in central nervous dysfunction. Neuropsychological tests have notable limitations, the primary one being that they are designed to pinpoint specific abnormalities (say, frontal lobe defects), but not to identify more subtle dysfunctions (such as those resulting from toxins affecting many areas of the brain).

Other psychological tests rely heavily on subjective interpretation, meaning that the same test may be interpreted very differently by two different psychologists. The Rorschach Inkblot Test, one of the most popular in psychology, is a good example. The test consists of ten inkblots, some black or gray and some colored, on cards. A patient is shown the cards one at a time and is asked to say what each card looks like. Supposedly, based on a patient's responses, a psychologist can tell whether he or she is "paranoid," "obsessive," or whatever. But to do so, the psychologist must decide whether a patient's responses are normal or abnormal—a completely subjective process. (Who is to say whether an inkblot should look like a crockpot or a cat—and what kind of training could possibly teach such wisdom?)

In *House of Cards,* psychology researcher Robyn Dawes explains how dangerous such tests can be when used to "diagnose" illness. At one point in his career, when he was still a believer in the power of the Rorschach, he tested a 16-year-old girl being held against her will in a hospital, for the "symptom" of dating an older man. All of the girl's answers on the Rorschach were routine, except when she said that card number eight looked like a bear (which, to most people at least, it doesn't). Dawes reported his findings in a staff meeting, and the head psychologist then asked the assembled staff members, "Does that look like a bear to you?" When everyone said no, Dawes says, the head psychologist "then 'explained why' the girl had said it looked like a bear: she had been hallucinating." Based on that one inkblot, the psychologist declared that the girl was schizophrenic—although, Dawes notes, she appeared mature, smart, and quite normal.

Needless to say, this is not a good way to "diagnose" brain dysfunction. Neither is any pen-and-paper test, including those used by neuropsychologists. Psychological tests can be useful in limited ways, but they should never be the sole basis for a diagnosis. C. Jagger and colleagues, in a recently published evaluation of a psychological test commonly used to "diagnose" dementia, pointed out the fallacy of relying on such tests. The researchers found that individuals who were over age 84, or belonged to lower social classes, or had visual impairments were at great risk of being mislabeled by the test.

Neither a psychologist nor a neuropsychologist has the capacity to make an assessment of the causes of symptoms, despite a knowledge of DSM terminology. Medical diagnosis is the province of the physician, who has the tools and expertise necessary to diagnose brain dysfunction by the process of differential diagnosis. I have tremendous respect for the work that social workers, psychologists, neuropsychologists, and counselors do; but, just as I don't claim to have the knowledge necessary to do their jobs well, I don't believe that they have the medical knowledge to do mine well. So, if your goal is to obtain a medical diagnosis, be sure you're seeing a *psychiatrist*—not a psychologist or counselor or social worker. And don't let titles fool you; be sure the "Doctor" in front of your doctor's name means M.D., not Ph.D.

After you have received an accurate diagnosis and any appropriate management for your condition, psychologists and social workers can play important roles in your recovery. Much psychotherapy, as I've noted, is provided by non-M.D. psychologists and social workers. And social workers can also guide you to helpful services, such as support groups and financial assistance.

When You See a Doctor, Be Assertive and Get Your Questions Answered

Do you frequently leave a doctor's office dissatisfied, because you didn't get answers to your questions or you felt intimidated by a doctor's superior, impatient attitude? If so, you're not alone. As Charles Inlander and colleagues point out, in *Medicine on Trial,*

> . . . doctors over recent generations have established the ground rules for patient behavior, especially regarding the patient's relationship to (and critique of) the doctor. Many of us are taught (or intuit) that it is not good form to play too active a role, never mind a contentious one. Questions to doctors should be polite and deferential, acknowledging their superior knowledge and the wisdom of experience. If we are irritated with the doctor's demeanor in any way or left with any uneasy feeling that something is not right in the care being given, we might save our gripes for relatives or friends.

In my opinion, such deference to doctors is a dangerous thing. Physicians who treat patients and their relatives brusquely or condescendingly—intimidating them into silence rather than encouraging them to offer input or ask questions—are far more likely to miss a diagnosis than those who listen carefully. This is as true in psychiatry as in other medical fields. Dawes, commenting on "the implicit principle that we shouldn't take seriously what a disturbed person has to say," notes that "there is absolutely no evidence that emotional distress necessarily implies incompetence or an inability to judge what is helping or hurting in an attempt to alleviate that distress." And even when a patient is too impaired to be a full participant in a psychiatric examination, his or her family members are not. They should be treated as valuable sources of information and enlightenment, nor as annoying interlopers or, worse, contributors to the patient's problems.

I don't expect my patients, or their family members, to hand me an accurate diagnosis—after all, that's my job—but I do recognize that they are in many ways more expert than I am. For instance, the mother of a hyperactive child knows far more than I do about her child's prenatal history, delivery complications, and early development. She knows whether her child chews on toys, wets the bed, grinds his or her teeth, has trouble with math, or gets carsick. Clues like these spark the initial questions that, in time, grow into a diagnosis. By combining a mother's expert knowledge of her individual child with my expert knowledge of medicine, we become a formidable diagnostic team. (This doesn't mean that I have to agree with all of her opinions about causation. It does mean, however, that I should treat them with respect.)

In this less-than-perfect world, however, you're likely to get an intimidating psychiatrist, or one who's too rushed to listen carefully, or one who dismisses your concerns and questions condescendingly. So be prepared. Read the "Patient's Bill of Rights for Psychiatric Treatment," on page 188, before you visit a psychiatrist's office. When you go for your appointment, take along a list of all the questions you want to ask, and don't leave until they're answered. Be assertive; remember that it's your health at stake, not the doctor's.

Also, if possible, take along a friend or relative who can stand up for you if necessary, can make sure your questions get asked and answered, and will accurately remember what happened at the visit— something that may be hard to do yourself if the visit is an

---

Patient's Bill of Rights for Psychiatric Treatment

- You have the right to a deductive differential diagnosis—no matter how much time it takes.
- You have the right to question your doctor, particularly if his or her "diagnosis" is based on DSM rather than on established medical diagnostic techniques.
- You have the right to obtain a second opinion—and as many subsequent opinions as you want.
- You have the right to be fully informed about your condition and your treatment.
- You have the right to disagree with a recommended treatment and to inquire about alternative treatments.
- You have the right to be fully informed about the risks and benefits of any medication prescribed for you.
- Your family members have the right, if you so choose, to be partners in your treatment.
- If you choose psychotherapy as part of your treatment, you have the right to terminate the therapy at any time without recrimination from your therapist.

---

emotional experience. (It is, incidentally, no crime to become emotional at the doctor's office, particularly when you are discussing something as frightening as a brain dysfunction.) And, as Inlander points out, "A third person in the examining room is also a not-so-subtle reminder to the doctor that he or she had better be on best behavior."

Don't Be Bamboozled by Jargon

It's critically important that you understand what your doctor tells you about your condition. If you don't understand your doctor's terminology, ask for a translation into simpler terms. Some physicians honestly forget that patients may not know what *dyskinetic* or *hypoplastic* means. Others may use big terms to impress their listeners. In either case, ask your physician to communicate with you in language you can understand. And request a written report afterward. (If your report includes test results, be sure to save them. Even normal test results may be handy, months or years later, as "baseline" records in case your medical condition changes.) I myself provide each patient with an audiotape of my concluding diagnostic conference.

Above all, don't be fooled by jargon—particularly psychoanalytic jargon—that's simply a fancy cover-up for a DSM label. Many patients seeking real diagnoses for their problems wind up falling for the convincing patter of psychoanalytically-oriented doctors. But psychoanalytic explanations, although they sound terribly erudite, are useless when it comes to treating brain disorders. Take this "diagnostic" information, from the *New Harvard Guide to Psychiatry* (1988 edition):

> In psychodynamic terms, anxiety is a sign of psychological conflict resulting from the threatened emergence into consciousness of forbidden, repressed mental contents. . . . What the individual fears is the escape from the prison house of the unconscious of aggressive and libidinal drives and their derivative emotions and fantasies.

Whew! That certainly sounds impressive, but it doesn't explain the anxiety attacks caused by medication errors, allergic reactions, hyperthyroidism, and dozens of other diagnosable and treatable disorders. Patients whose anxiety stems from such disorders aren't going to feel better if they spend thousands of dollars letting their fantasies escape from the "prison house of the unconscious"; they're only going to feel angry and cheated when they find out that treatments based on such theories are worthless.

So keep your resolve. Remind yourself, before going to the psychiatrist, that you're going to get a real diagnosis. Don't be impressed by any substitutes, no matter what fancy language your doctor uses. And don't leave the doctor's office until your doctor has told you, in plain English, what's wrong with you and what can be done about it.

If You're over Sixty, or under Twelve, Beware!

As I've already mentioned, women are more likely than men to be misdiagnosed by psychiatrists. But children and seniors are also at particularly high risk for the label-and-drug DSM syndrome.

CHILDREN

Millions of children with diagnosable disorders are labeled as having "hyperactivity" or "attention deficit disorder." But there's another DSM label catching up with these two in popularity among child psychiatrists: posttraumatic stress disorder (PTSD). The current belief—which, I might add, doesn't seem to be supported by any good evidence—is that normal children, exposed to even minor traumas, often develop severe, long-term behavioral and emotional symptoms. This belief has led to the nontreatment or mistreatment of thousands of anxious, irritable, learning disabled, aggressive, or perfectly normal children.

One of them, Paul, recently came to see me. A bright African American child with an engaging (but somewhat toothless) grin, Paul had fallen off an amusement park ride and cut his ear severely. His wound required several stitches and an overnight stay in a hospital, but it had healed completely by the time he started first grade several months later. However, when Paul began experiencing problems at school and at home—including tantrums, destructive behaviors, headaches, and dizziness—one of his doctors suggested that a psychiatrist examine him for PTSD.

But Paul didn't have posttraumatic stress disorder. In fact, like most young kids, he'd experienced only minor, temporary anxiety following his accident. When I asked him about his accident, he had the normal childhood reaction: his eyes lit up, and he said, "You wanna see my scar?" Paul was clearly much less traumatized by his accident than his mother, who was concerned that it might scar him for life.

After a careful history revealed symptoms prior to his accident, it was clear to me that Paul's problems started long before he fell off the carnival ride. I found, upon further examination, that Paul had a significant hearing defect, a mildly elevated lead level, and evidence of a parasitic infection. None of these problems, obviously, had anything to do with "posttraumatic stress."

Giving children like Paul a "diagnosis" of PTSD does them a terrible disservice, because most of these children have disorders that will continue to interfere with their lives and their education if not addressed. Paul, for instance, would have fallen further and further behind in class—even though he was brighter than most of his classmates—simply because his hearing defect and lead poisoning would have gone unnoticed.

SENIOR CITIZENS

When you become a senior citizen, your risk of both suffering a brain dysfunction and being misdiagnosed increases exponentially. Here's why.

- *Your body is different.* As you age, your metabolism slows down. Your immune system becomes less efficient at fighting off invading bacteria and viruses. Your blood vessels become harder, your muscles shrink, and your heart doesn't pump as much blood. These changes aren't "abnormal"; they simply mean that you may be more susceptible to infections, reduced blood flow to the brain, nutritional deficiencies, and other risk factors for brain dysfunction.
- *You're probably taking more medications.* At the very time when your body is most susceptible to medication-related problems (primarily because of slower metabolism), you're most likely to be taking multiple powerful drugs. Seniors take more drugs, more often, than any other segment of the population. And the drugs they take—heart medications,

blood pressure medications, sleeping pills, and so on—are those most likely to interfere with brain function.

- *Your standard of living may be lower.* Many seniors, getting by on small fixed incomes, live in older housing (which, as I've noted, increases their risk of carbon monoxide poisoning); eat poorly, often causing nutritional deficiencies; and let medical problems slide, rather than having them treated when they first occur. All of these factors can increase the risk of brain dysfunction.
- *If you're over sixty, and particularly if you're over eighty, your symptoms are likely to be written off as "normal" signs of aging.* Doctors are just now beginning to realize that extensive memory loss, despondency, fatigue, and similar symptoms *aren't* normal parts of the aging process but signs of disease (and psychiatry, generally the last medical field to find out the latest news, is well behind in this area). Thus, as physician Sidney Wolfe and colleagues note, in *Best Pills, Worst Pills,* confusion or memory loss in a young patient will be viewed with concern by a physician, while "the same symptoms in an older person, especially if they develop more slowly, are often dismissed with a familiar remark, 'Well, he (or she) is just growing old, what do you expect?'"

When psychiatrists *do* realize that an older patient has a serious brain dysfunction, they are all too likely to label it as Alzheimer's or some other form of incurable dementia. Many patients *do* suffer from Alzheimer's and other dementias; but thousands more, who are labeled as having dementia, are actually suffering from problems that can be corrected. Studies suggest, in fact, that up to 60 percent of patients tentatively labeled as having "dementia" actually have treatable and reversible disorders.

A typical case of brain dysfunction misdiagnosed as dementia—cited by Siegfried Kra, in *Aging Myths*—involved a well-known and well-liked judge who was a friend of Kra's family. "My parents first noted a change in his behavior when they played bridge together one day," Kra says. "The judge was unable to recall the cards and then became angry." As time went on, the judge began crying or laughing at odd times, and became abusive and demanding. The court stopped giving him cases, and he was arrested twice for lewd behavior. Several psychiatrists labeled this gentleman as having "brain degeneration," and said that there was no help for his condition.

Luckily, Kra says, the man's wife was unwilling to accept their verdict. She took him to another psychiatrist who discovered that the arteries to the judge's brain were clogged with cholesterol. Surgery to remove the cholesterol plaques led to an almost complete recovery, and Kra reports that the judge is "still alive and very much an active person."

A similar case of "incurable" dementia with a simple and treatable underlying cause is related by psychiatrist Abraham Twerski, in *Who Says You're Neurotic?* The patient, a 71-year-old man who had always been in good health, suddenly began exhibiting dramatic mental deterioration. His memory became very poor, he developed a shuffling gait, and he became apathetic and was unable to do simple chores such as balancing a checkbook.

The man's doctors gave him a DSM "diagnosis" of incurable dementia. He continued to gradually deteriorate—just as they'd predicted—until, one day, he was unable to get out of bed. His wife, believing he'd had a stroke, arranged for hospitalization. While he was in the hospital, he wet the bed several times, prompting the staff to call in a urologist, who diagnosed prostate problems and recommended surgery. The prostate surgery—seemingly unrelated to the man's senility—caused a remarkable change in his behavior. His confusion and despondency cleared, his memory became as good as ever, and his other symptoms of senility vanished completely.

It turns out, Twerski explains, that well before the patient's mental symptoms developed, he had begun wetting the bed (a symptom of his developing prostate problem). The man was so embarrassed by the bedwetting, and so afraid it would happen again, that he fought going to sleep. "The mental symptoms he was manifesting," Twerski says, "were caused by sleep deprivation." A good physical examination would have uncovered both the man's prostate trouble and his lack of sleep, and saved him and his family much grief.

There are two lessons to be learned from such cases: (1) emotional and behavioral symptoms aren't "normal" signs of aging, and (2) such symptoms, no matter how abnormal or frightening, usually aren't signs of Alzheimer's disease or other untreatable dementias. In the majority of cases, such symptoms have diagnosable causes, treatments, and cures.

Because these lessons are so important, I'm ending this section with one more story about a "demented" patient who wasn't demented at all. Her name was Deborah, and her family brought her to see me because they were convinced that she suffered from Alzheimer's disease. When I'd first seen the woman a few years earlier, for a minor complaint, she'd been elegantly dressed and meticulous, and had spoken with a cultivated Boston accent that I suspected was somewhat "put on." But when her family brought her in the second time, she was unwashed and drooling. She picked her nose in front of me, and when I administered a pinprick test, she swore at me in a very un-Bostonian accent—and then kicked me! The cause of Deborah's startling change turned out to be not Alzheimer's, but carbon monoxide poisoning caused by a faulty pilot light on the gas heater in her new apartment.

Maybe Your Disorder Is Incurable/Maybe It Isn't

Dementia isn't the only label that frequently covers up a treatable disorder. Most psychiatrists also throw in the towel after labeling patients as having antisocial personality disorder, learning disabilities, pervasive developmental disorder, or a number of other disorders considered to be untreatable (except through special education or psychotherapy). Schizophrenia, in particular, is considered by most psychiatrists to be incurable, and patients or family members who go from doctor to doctor seeking help are thought of as being "in denial." Hyperactivity, too, is considered to be a lifelong disorder that can be masked by medication but not cured.

It's true that a large number of people labeled as "schizophrenic"—perhaps the vast majority—can't yet be accurately diagnosed and cured. But a surprising number can. After all, the millions of patients labeled as schizophrenic actually suffer from a variety of disorders; their symptoms may be caused by anything from incurable brain damage to readily treatable drug reactions, infections, or metabolic abnormalities. And when the problem is hyperactivity, I believe that cures should be the rule—not the exception. "Learning disabilities" and "pervasive developmental disorders" also are labels that can conceal dozens of diagnosable, treatable, and sometimes curable brain disorders.

I contend that virtually no "mental" disorder is incurable in 100 percent of cases. *In the absence of brain scans showing actual physical damage, there is no basis for saying that a disorder is incurable simply because it qualifies for a DSM label.* It is immoral to give up on a patient when there is no evidence of irreparable brain damage. Dysfunction, in the absence of damage, is potentially reversible.

Many people *do* have untreatable, incurable brain disorders; you may be one of them. If you receive a diagnosis of "incurable" illness, I suggest that you accept that the prognosis may be correct—and prepare accordingly—but bear in mind that it may be *in*correct. Don't spend every minute of your time, or every penny of your money, frantically running from doctor to doctor, but *do* investigate any promising new leads. Find out whether any medical facilities in the country (or outside of it) are doing state-of-the-art research on your disorder. Keep abreast of the medical literature and see whether other physicians know something your doctor doesn't. (This isn't a slap at doctors. No single human being, no matter how dedicated and intelligent, could know everything there is to know about the brain.)

Don't be surprised, however, if your physician (particularly if he or she is a psychiatrist) becomes angry when you suggest that your "incurable" disease may in fact be curable. Some doctors react poorly to having their opinions challenged. That's their problem, not yours. (I always tell my patients, honestly, if I believe their suggestions aren't medically valid, and explain why, but I don't get angry at them for exploring every possible avenue. In their position, I would too.) If your doctor gives up before you're ready to, find another doctor.

There is, incidentally, no crime in "doctor-shopping." I'm always amazed at how many doctors describe a patient who seeks out the opinions of several specialists as "a pathetic individual who can't accept reality." I've successfully diagnosed and treated patients who had been to literally dozens of doctors without obtaining relief. Perhaps some patients I wasn't able to diagnose and treat continued their search and found help elsewhere. If patients aren't willing to give up hope, who am I to blame them?

Another piece of advice: if your psychiatrist (or any other physician) diagnoses an incurable disorder, based on laboratory test results, have the tests readministered at least once—and preferably twice. Human error or equipment error often leads to erroneous test results, and many an "incurable" patient has written a will and purchased a burial plot, only to learn that the lab results were wrong.

One more thing: even if you do have a disorder we can't yet cure, don't let your doctor blame every new symptom you develop on the disorder. In many cases, new symptoms are a sign of a completely unrelated problem that can be diagnosed and treated. A good example involved a retarded child who suddenly began striking himself in the face savagely, causing severe injury to his face and teeth. Psychiatrists assured the family that this was a common symptom in the severely retarded (which it is), but failed to consider the idea that the behavior might stem from some other cause. It did: the family later discovered that the child was suffering from a severely abscessed tooth. Because he was mute, his only way of communicating his distress was through a dramatic physical display. By the time his true problem was discovered, the child had spent several months on powerful psychotropic drugs that had caused additional behavioral symptoms. I've heard of similar patients whose self-injury, aggression, or other behavior problems resulted from urinary tract infections, ear infections, or bowel impaction, and a recent report has linked severe eye-poking in some children labeled as autistic to a calcium deficiency readily treated with supplements.

Remember: one diagnosis (even if it *is* a diagnosis, and not a DSM label) doesn't preclude another, and people with incurable disorders can, just like the rest of us, develop additional, treatable medical problems. As noted neurologist Sir Francis Walshe once said, "Many psychiatrists . . . tend to forget, if a patient's history contains the material of a psychiatric explanation, that this does not render him immune to all the ills that flesh is heir to, nor exclude the presence of one or more of them."

Never Accept a Drug Unquestioningly

There are times—although they're few and far between—when drugs are a legitimate treatment for a brain dysfunction. But it's *never* appropriate for a physician to prescribe drugs—particularly dangerous psychotropic drugs—on the basis of a DSM label, without conducting a deductive differential diagnosis. Remember the cardinal rule of medicine: treatment comes *after* diagnosis, not before.

Remember, also, that few doctors have more than a basic and superficial training in pharmacology, and most are too harried to keep up with the literature on effects and side effects of drugs. Many doctors rely far too much on information provided by drug companies, which inflate the values and downplay the dangers of their products. So leaving your medication decisions solely in the hands of your doctor isn't always advisable.

If your physician, after performing a deductive differential diagnosis, does conclude that a psychotropic drug is appropriate, ask why. Ask whether the drug is being used to treat a disorder, or merely to mask symptoms—and, if the latter (which is usually the case), ask yourself whether the risks of the drug outweigh its benefits. And be sure you *know* all of the risks; ask both your doctor and your pharmacist about the drug's potential side effects, and then look it up in the *Physician's Desk Reference* (PDR) or one of the many drug guides available in bookstores and libraries. (Be aware, however, that the PDR lists even the most rare side effects. Just about every drug, including the relatively safe ones, sounds pretty scary in the PDR. So, when reading the PDR listings, focus on side effects listed as common. Or select one of the many pocketbook drug guides on the market; these tend to give you a better picture of the real risks of each drug.) If you have access to computer literature searches, run a search on the name of the drug and see what current research has to say about its efficacy and safety. Learn about any potential risks of mixing the medication with other drugs (either prescription or over-the-counter) or with alcohol. Find out what the standard dosage of the drug is, and if your dosage is significantly higher, ask your doctor why. In addition, ask your doctor to spell out the name of the drug he or she is prescribing, and the dosage, and write this information down yourself. Later, when you pick up your prescription, verify that the information on the bottle matches what you've written down.

If all of this double-checking sounds a bit paranoid, consider the studies suggesting that up to a third of all hospital admissions are for complications from treatment—usually drug treatment—by a doctor. Often, such reactions occur because physicians prescribe drugs about which they know very little. But even doctors who know a great deal about drug effects and side effects may not pass sufficient information on to patients; one study found that, more than three-fourths of the time, doctors failed to give their patients clear instructions about how drugs should be taken.

When you get a correctly written prescription and clear instructions from the physician, you're still not home free, because pharmacy errors happen more often than you'd think. Half of the druggists responding to one poll said that they had dispensed incorrect prescriptions because they couldn't read doctors' handwriting. (And overworked pharmacists at one large drugstore chain went on strike in June 1990, complaining that their heavy workload caused an unacceptable risk of errors.) If you are taking psychotropic drugs, which are powerful and very dangerous medications, even minor errors or miscommunications can be deadly.

A few more cautions are in order:

1. *Be especially careful about any drugs (particularly psychotropic drugs) prescribed while you're in a hospital.* If your symptoms make it impossible for you to handle this responsibility, family members should do it for you. A recent article in *Drug Topics,* a newsletter for pharmacists, notes that "in an average U.S. hospital, every hour of every day, 60 patients are given either the wrong dosage or the wrong medication." The article notes that poor handwriting and carelessness can lead to lethal drug mistakes. (Even a more conservative estimate I've heard—360 medication errors per day for an average-size hospital—is hardly reassuring.) I am not being facetious when I tell my patients that the most dangerous place in the community is the hospital.

2. *Doctors frequently increase the dosage of an ineffective medication, figuring that "more is better."* But in the case of psychotropic drugs, higher dosages may be no more effective than lower dosages and can increase your risk of serious side effects. If increasing a dose does not help, or if you begin experiencing new symptoms, tell your physician immediately—or ask a second doctor for an opinion about your medications. And never increase your dosage on your own; the "window of safety" for some psychotropic medications is very small.

3. *If you are taking psychotropic drugs, do NOT stop taking them without consulting your physician.* Reducing the dosage of psychotropic drugs too suddenly can result in serious or even life-threatening withdrawal effects. A doctor can tell you how to safely taper off medications.

4. *Beware of "polypharmacy."* Too often, physicians prescribe psychotropic drugs that create side effects, and then administer yet more drugs to counter the side effects of the original drugs. After a while, it's impossible to tell which symptoms are caused by the patient's underlying ailment and which are caused by the drugs given to treat it.

5. *Be suspicious of newspaper ads that offer free testing for Alzheimer's or other disorders as part of a drug trial.* Generally, such ads are simply a means of rounding up human guinea pigs for tests of new drugs that are of questionable value and safety. The "free tests" are generally pen-and-paper psychological tests, or quick evaluations by doctors, neither of which can accurately diagnose brain dysfunction.

6. *Don't assume that a prescription for Prozac or benzodiazepines or antidepressants means that your doctor is doing his or her job.* We've become too accustomed to the idea that every successful visit to a doctor's office ends with a prescription; or, as author Kathryn Watterson puts it, we've bought into the idea of "the prescription as a lollipop." See for yourself how pervasive this attitude is: next time you go to the doctor, tell your friends where you've been and see how many of them say, "What did you get?" The idea that you have to "get something" at the end of every doctor's appointment is not only a dangerous idea but an expensive one, given the astonishingly high cost of many modern medications. If you accept a prescription, do it for a good reason—not just because it's handed to you.

7. *Never allow your psychiatrist to medicate a nonsymptom.* As I've noted, psychiatrists are increasingly "treating" perfectly healthy people with drugs that can alter brain chemistry and

cause serious long-term brain dysfunction. This is an extremely dangerous experiment, both morally and medically, and my advice is to resist being a part of it. Be skeptical of TV reports that Prozac can control your overshopping or overeating. Don't expect designer personality drugs to save your love life, overcome your natural inhibitions, or cure your job dissatisfaction. And if you suffer a loss or trauma, work through it; don't attempt to mask your grief with drugs that will only delay coming to terms with reality. Nobody is supposed to have either a perfect personality or a perfect life, and attempting to create either one chemically is dangerous and unethical.

Don't Let a Psychologist Prescribe Your Medication

Given the dangers of psychotropic drugs, which I've discussed throughout this book, it seems obvious that the power to prescribe these drugs should be carefully controlled. Instead, efforts are being made to *reduce* control over who is allowed to prescribe these drugs. These efforts stem, again, from the mistaken idea that listing symptoms and attaching a DSM label to them—something a psychologist can do as easily as a psychiatrist—is comparable to "diagnosing" a disease.

This fallacy in thinking has led to a growing movement to allow psychologists to prescribe psychotropic medications. If you're a member of the military, or live on a Native American reservation, psychologists are already allowed by law to prescribe psychotropic drugs for you. Several states are considering extending prescription privileges to psychologists; this would allow any patient to obtain a prescription for "depression" or "anxiety" straight from a Ph.D.

What's the drawback? Unlike psychiatrists, who are medical doctors, psychologists are not trained in the science of medical diagnosis; their expertise lies in testing (for instance, administering IQ tests) and in statistical analysis. A psychologist is no more likely to diagnose leptospirosis, or pernicious anemia, or brain tumors, than your barber is.

"To prescribe medications," AMA president John Tupper has noted, "the person needs a knowledge of biochemistry, physiology and pharmacology. Along with that, [the person needs] clinical experience in the management of patients and drug therapy." In other words, the person should be a medical doctor. Psychiatrists, although their diagnostic skills are somewhat atrophied, have the medical background necessary to diagnose and treat disease and to prescribe appropriate medications. Psychologists, although skilled in their own field, can't diagnose brain disease or the causes of dysfunction. They can only learn to apply DSM cookbook labels based on symptoms.

So be extremely careful about accepting a prescription from an M.D., but *refuse* altogether to accept one from a psychologist. And never allow your psychiatrist to prescribe a drug based solely on a psychologist's recommendations—an all-too-common practice.

If You Choose to Participate in Psychotherapy, Choose a Therapist with Whom You Feel Comfortable

As I've noted, therapy can be helpful, not in treating underlying brain dysfunction but in easing the emotional fallout this dysfunction causes. But therapy can, in some cases, cause significant harm. So if you decide to see a therapist, be a smart consumer. Don't accept a referral for therapy until you've received an accurate diagnosis—not a DSM label, but a real diagnosis—and treatment for any medical conditions. Find out up front what type of therapy a potential therapist practices, and avoid any therapies that focus entirely on negative emotions and past traumas. And once you're in therapy, give your therapist a chance; but if, after a dozen or so sessions, you are dissatisfied or extremely uncomfortable, or feel the therapist is pushing a personal agenda rather than listening to you, leave and find another therapist.

Leaving therapy isn't always as easy as it sounds. Jerrold Maxmen, a therapist and author of *The New Psychiatry*, comments that his psychiatric colleagues often are critical of patients who terminate therapy without mutual agreement. "I'd guess that 10 to 20 percent of all psychotherapies end with the psychiatrist's full endorsement," he says. "Another 10 to 20 percent of the time psychiatrists feel ambivalent about the patient's terminating. The rest of the time psychiatrists think it's a lousy decision." Nonmutual terminations, he says, tend to be blamed on patients' "acting out," "masochism," "need to fail," or "negativism"—rarely on the therapists themselves.

Maxmen adds that therapists sometimes manipulate patients into staying in therapy by making them feel guilty or uncomfortable, or by insinuating that they are trying to avoid facing their problems. Pressure tactics like these should not dissuade you from leaving if you have given the therapy a fair chance and have seen that it is useless or counterproductive. Remember: the minute you walk out the door, your involvement with a therapist is over, and you don't have to worry about hurt feelings. Remember as well that psychotherapy is *not* a medical treatment; thus, changing therapists is not like walking out of a hospital against medical advice, but more like leaving a bad relationship that's not working out.

This is especially important to remember if you become involved in negative therapies such as repressed memory therapy, which I discussed earlier. Such therapies often use techniques not dissimilar from brainwashing methods to keep clients from leaving. If you suspect you're stuck in this kind of situation, get out and seek more appropriate help. There are many forms of therapy, and you'll probably find one that's right for you—or discover that you don't need therapy at all.

If you encounter therapies that you feel are ineffective or destructive, let your psychiatrist—if he or she referred you—know about it. Psychiatrists should be held accountable not only for the therapies they themselves practice, but also for the therapies they recommend. (Telling your psychiatrist that you've left therapy, however, could result in yet another DSM "diagnosis": Code V15.81, "Noncompliance With Treatment." This label can be applied to any patient leaving therapy for "decisions based on personal value judgments or religious or cultural beliefs about the advantages and disadvantages of the proposed treatment"—in other words, virtually any patient who believes that a therapy isn't helpful!)

Do Your Homework: Read Up on Your Condition

As John Steinbeck once noted, "The medical profession is unconsciously irritated by lay knowledge." Doctors, and psychiatrists in particular, tend to dislike patients who have diagnosed themselves based on advice they have seen on TV programs, or articles in popular magazines. It's true that a little knowledge is a dangerous thing, and that most diagnoses based on magazine articles or TV shows are worth about what you paid for them. Remember that any symptom can have hundreds of causes; for instance, your neighbor's twitch might be Bell's palsy, while yours might be Tourette's syndrome—or merely a minor nerve irritation.

It's true, also, that the more popular the medium, the less likely it is that the information you're getting from it is accurate. Because TV talk show hosts, news anchors, and TV "health correspondents" generally know little more about medicine than the lay public does, much of the information they give you is incomplete, misleading, or just plain wrong. For instance, a popular TV news show recently conducted a Medicare/Medicaid exposé that included an interview with an elderly, arthritic woman in Florida, whose doctor had ordered a syphilis test for her. The woman was appalled at the suggestion that she could have syphilis at her age. The reporter was shocked as well, and insinuated that the doctor was intentionally abusing the Medicare system. But the fact is, I most likely would have ordered the same test. Syphilis contracted in a patient's early years frequently hides in the body until decades later, when it can cause arthritis, brain dysfunctions, and a host of other puzzling symptoms. Even in later stages, it can be treated—often saving patients years of pain.

But while a little knowledge about medicine can be dangerous, particularly if that knowledge comes from poorly qualified sources, no knowledge at all is far more risky. A psychiatrist isn't going to tell you, in an hour-long visit, everything you need to know about your condition. (And a DSM-oriented psychiatrist may not tell you *anything* you need to know.) So learn as much as you can on your own—but seek out accurate sources. One of the best sources of up-to-date, accurate information is current medical journals, available either on computer networks (for a fee) or from the library (for free). If you live near a university, you can generally use the campus library even if you are not a student. Universities with medical schools are the best source of information, but libraries at most universities carry a wide range of medical journals.

And don't shy away completely from popular magazine articles about "mental" disorders. Friends of mine have sent me dozens of quite good articles, from *Redbook, Ladies Home Journal,* and similar magazines, about psychiatric misdiagnosis of thyroid disorders, infections, cancer, and other diseases. You shouldn't try to diagnose yourself based on such articles, but they can sometimes offer valuable information. Another resource is computer bulletin boards, which can put you in touch with other patients suffering from similar disorders. These sources can offer a wealth of information on good doctors—and sometimes help steer you away from bad ones.

*　*　*

This chapter may have given you the impression that it's difficult to find good help for psychiatric symptoms. Unfortunately, that impression is largely correct. But it's not impossible to find good medical care, if you're willing to be assertive and invest some time and money in the search for a psychiatrist who knows the difference between DSM and diagnosis, and understands the limitations of both psychotropic drugs and psychotherapy. My hope is that, as more psychiatrists and patients come forward to challenge the DSM-based system of nondiagnosis and nontreatment, the search will become easier.

So don't give up. There *are* psychiatrists who are trained in the art of differential diagnosis, who listen to their patients, and who are interested in treating the real causes of brain dysfunction rather than masking them with dangerous medications or prescribing ineffective therapies. No matter how many DSM labels and nondiagnoses you get, I encourage you to keep looking. Remember that almost all of the successful case histories I've talked about in this book involved patients who previously had been misdiagnosed; they eventually found help, and, with persistence and luck, so will you.

In doing so, you may be part of the next great revolution in psychiatry—the revolution that forces psychiatry to become a true medical profession that diagnoses and treats disorders rather than labeling their symptoms and masking their causes. I believe that by demanding proper care and by refusing to settle for DSM nondiagnoses or "managed care" or unnecessary drugs or misguided therapies, patients can play a tremendous role in guiding psychiatry into a new era of patient-oriented, scientifically sound medicine.

CHAPTER 8

"But I'm Not a Patient!"

Why You Still Need to Worry

Depending on [one psychiatric or psychological] expert's opinion, an individual may be confined to a mental institution, receive huge monetary awards, obtain custody of a child, or lose his or her life.

David Faust and Jay Ziskin,
in *Science*

The psychiatrist is the most important nongovernmental decision maker in modern life.

Jonas Robitscher, M.D.,
in *The Powers of Psychiatry*

As a physician, I've focused in this book on the medical consequences of DSM. Unfortunately, DSM can have a serious impact on your life *even if you never suffer from a brain dysfunction*. The manual's effects are felt far outside doctors' offices—in homes, business offices, courtrooms, and jails. DSM can be used to determine your fitness as a parent, your ability to do a job, even your right to support a particular political party. It can be used to keep a criminal in jail or to release a murderer back into society. It can be used to invalidate your will, to break your legal contracts, or to deny you the right to marry without a court's permission. If giving that much power to one book sounds scary, it is. But it's no exaggeration.

Here are some aspects of your personal life that can be affected by DSM psychiatry.

Your Job

If you want to know how powerful a DSM label can be, ask medical researcher Margaret Jensvold, a former employee at the National Institutes of Mental Health (NIMH). After complaining about harassment by male coworkers, she was sent to a psychiatrist, also employed by NIMH, who labeled her as having "self-defeating personality disorder." Shortly afterward, her fellowship at NIMH was terminated. She later sued NIMH for sexual discrimination, and won (after which she suggested that her label be changed to "self-empowering personality"). In the very next update of DSM-IV, the category of "self-defeating personality disorder" was eliminated—meaning that Jensvold may have lost her job because of a label that didn't even exist a few years later.

"People had predicted that if [self-defeating personality disorder] was in the DSM, women would be blamed for their own victimization," Jensvold told the *Los Angeles Times Magazine*, "and that's just what they were doing to me."

Fortunately, under the Americans with Disabilities Act (ADA), it's now harder to fire an employee based on arbitrary or politically motivated DSM labels. Unfortunately, this same law has led to the opposite problem: the inability of an employer to *fire* an employee for absenteeism, poor performance, or even kleptomania, because a psychiatrist has categorized the employee's behavior as a DSM-approved "disability." *Reason* magazine recently reported the case of an insurance firm employee who, after undergoing repressed memory therapy, became sad and embittered, started wearing black regularly, and began missing work on a regular basis. After about eight months of her aberrant behavior, her employer fired her—only to be socked with a lawsuit under the ADA because the woman claimed she was "depressed" and therefore was protected under the law. And the *Employee Relations Law Journal* recently noted that employees with DSM labels such as "histrionic personality disorder" or "narcissistic personality disorder" can be protected under the law—meaning that the incredibly self-centered jerk who takes advantage of everyone in the office, or the melodramatic employee who throws a potted plant at the boss when she complains about a missed deadline, is suffering from a "disability" and should not be held accountable. Such claims aren't rare; in fact, discrimination cases based on alleged psychiatric disability are one of the most common categories of complaints under the ADA.

If a DSM label itself isn't enough to get an employee permanently protected as "disabled," there's always iatrogenic (doctor-caused) psychiatric disability. Many employees are now being labeled as disabled, and therefore protected under the ADA, because they have experienced (or claim to have experienced) bizarre reactions to psychotropic drugs prescribed by DSM-oriented physicians. The *American Spectator* recently cited a case in which an employee was fired from GTE Data Services after he was caught robbing purses in the office. The employee sued GTE, claiming that a bad reaction to Prozac had caused a mental disability that led him to steal. A federal judge agreed, saying that GTE should have tried to find some "reasonable accommodation" for the man's "disability." And a professor of philosophy at Boston University sued the university after he was fired for allegedly sexually assaulting a female professor. Although he denies the charges, the professor also claims to have been mentally disabled by prescription antidepressants and tranquilizers that "loosened his inhibitions," and says his firing violates the ADA.

Thus, if you're a business owner, DSM can hit you hard in the pocketbook. Virtually any incompetent, hostile, dishonest, or slovenly employee can find a psychiatrist who'll give him or her a DSM label—or a drug whose side effects will cause a "disability." And if you try to fire the employee after that, you're likely to find yourself in court.

What about employees whose behavior problems are caused by real brain dysfunctions? As I've demonstrated, DSM-oriented psychiatrists rarely diagnose and correct such problems. Thus, employers pay thousands of dollars for medical insurance that covers the nondiagnosis and mismanagement of their employees' "psychiatric" disorders—and then are forced to keep these employees on the job indefinitely, in spite of bizarre or even dangerous behavior, after the same psychiatrists pronounce them incurable and thus permanently "disabled." It's a situation Kafka could have appreciated.

Your Legal Rights

These days, psychiatrists seem to outnumber lawyers in America's courts. In particular, psychiatrists are increasingly being used in civil cases such as competency hearings and custody disputes, where their power to determine the fate of individuals based solely on DSM "diagnoses" is often frightening.

DSM-IV does contain a disclaimer that "there are significant risks that diagnostic information will be misused or misunderstood" in legal settings, and the manual's authors state that DSM labels, in and of themselves, are not a sufficient basis for legally determining competence, criminal responsibility, or disability. These warnings, however, have largely fallen on deaf ears—as anyone who has been a party in a court proceeding involving psychiatric expert witnesses knows all too well.

A typical example of the abuses of psychiatry in the courtroom, cited in *Money* magazine, involved a 104-year-old Pittsburgh man who threatened to leave his two daughters less money in his will than his sons. His daughters, unhappy over his decision, petitioned the court to have him declared incompetent. According to *Money*, a psychiatrist hired by the daughters spent less than one hour with the women's father, and then declared that he was suffering from dementia—a disorder that could not possibly be accurately diagnosed, by anyone, in 50 minutes. A second psychiatrist who examined the man (apparently about as quickly) ruled that he was quite competent. Nevertheless, a judge ruled that the gentleman was incompetent, based on the first psychiatrist's testimony. As for the psychiatrists, *Money* reports that they walked away with $7,500 each—paid out of the elderly man's funds.

Maybe this man did have dementia. Maybe he didn't. The point is that neither psychiatrist could say, based on a brief interview, whether the DSM label of dementia was correct. A lengthy evaluation and a variety of studies are needed to establish whether a patient has a brain dysfunction, and, if so, whether it is true dementia or one of hundreds of other disorders that mimic dementia. Apparently no such studies were done by either psychiatric "expert" in this case, despite the seriousness of the issue being decided. Unfortunately, such curbside DSM diagnoses are becoming standard fare in competency hearings.

A similar example of psychiatric power and its consequences, cited by Stuart Kirk and Herb Kutchins in *The Selling of DSM*, involved a wealthy and influential man judged by a court to be incompetent and stripped of his voting rights, his ability to manage his own money, and his right to marry without the permission of a court. The reason? The man's parents disapproved of his support of controversial politician Lyndon LaRouche. Fearing that he would give his inheritance to LaRouche's political party, they found a psychiatrist willing to testify that their son suffered from schizoaffective disorder and had supported LaRouche "as an expression of his mental illness." Now, whatever one thinks of Lyndon LaRouche, supporting his political party is not, in and of itself, a sign of "mental illness." The fact that a psychiatrist could label it as such, and thus contribute to a court's decision to have this man stripped of his rights and property, shows how dangerous the combination of DSM and the American legal system can be.

Parents who have been involved in divorce and custody battles already know the power of DSM in a courtroom. That's because more and more custody battles are turning into duels between high-priced psychiatric and psychological expert witnesses wielding the DSM. DSM labels can be the basis for establishing that a parent is "dependent" or "histrionic" or "avoidant," and thus not fit to raise a child. They can be used to "diagnose" a child as having conduct disorder or oppositional defiant disorder as a result of faulty child-rearing practices by one parent or the other.

They can be used to decide who gets custody, who gets visitation rights, how long visitation should be and where it should take place. In short, DSM labels give psychiatrists the authority to make decisions that will affect children and their parents for years to come.

Unfortunately, these decisions are often based on quick interviews paid for by lawyers looking for "diagnoses" favorable to their clients and harmful to their clients' spouses. Stephen Herman and Alan Levy note, in *Children Today,* that "when a clinician begins an evaluation with only one option in mind—that of single-parent custody—he automatically places himself in a position of having to find a 'good' parent and a 'bad' one." Because DSM makes it easy to label any person on earth as disturbed or dysfunctional in some way, placing blame is not hard to do. Not surprisingly, psychiatrists generally find the parent for whom they are testifying to be more stable mentally than the parent who isn't paying them.

Even more unfortunately, because the price tag for such expert witnesses is often high, the parent with the fewest financial resources is the one most likely to be labeled as unfit. Psychiatrists, for instance, generally charge a minimum of $500 (and sometimes up to $2,000) per day to testify. "Custody cases are a real problem," one public lawyer said recently. "It's just hard to afford the clinical psychologists or physicians who will testify that the poor parent is competent."

In *Mothers on Trial,* Phyllis Chesler offers a chilling example of how a parent with money can use psychiatric experts to deny custody to a less well-to-do parent. A woman filed for divorce from her wealthy husband after he had lived apart from her and her children, with a mistress, for years. The wife was awarded child support and alimony, as well as custody. The husband, however, refused to pay the money he owed. Several years later, when he was more than $70,000 in arrears on these court-ordered payments, he sued for custody. His charge? That the wife's "obsession" with collecting the alimony and child support owed to her made her "mentally unfit." Chesler notes, "One psychiatrist assured the judge that, in his *psychiatric* opinion, [the mother] was receiving enough money." Based on the testimony of several psychiatrists hired by the husband, custody was granted to the man because of his spouse's "obsessional" disorder—that is, her insistence on receiving the alimony and child support payments a previous court had deemed were legally due her.

Even when money isn't involved, the testimony of psychiatric and psychological "experts" at custody hearings can be dangerous. That's because court-appointed professionals—who tend to have less training and expertise than other practitioners—are often called on to render judgments as to the mental fitness or unfitness of parties in custody cases. And these parties are often "diagnosed" by psychologists rather than psychiatrists. What do the psychologists use to make such "diagnoses," when they aren't medical doctors and can't perform any physical evaluations? The primary tool in their diagnostic arsenal is—what else?—the DSM.

The dangers of DSM "diagnoses" being administered by overworked and often ill-qualified employees of the court are well illustrated by another case cited by Chesler. A woman's ex-husband sued for custody even though he had tried to strangle her and had kidnapped her children. The woman was labeled by a court-appointed psychiatrist as being "paranoid" because of her reaction to the man's violence, and custody was granted to her ex-husband.

Your Protection from Criminals

Should a rapist be paroled? Has a child molester been "cured"? Was a killer insane at the time he strangled his wife? Is a murderer still dangerous, or can he be released into society? Questions like these are routinely decided by mental health professionals—generally, psychiatrists and psychologists—testifying as "expert witnesses." Their testimony is based on the premise that DSM labels are valid and can be used to analyze past and current mental health, as well as to predict future behavior.

This premise is entirely false. There is strong evidence that the psychiatric and psychological expert witnesses who have so much influence over juries are no more "expert" in making judgments about the mental health and future behavior of individuals than anyone else. In a *Science* article that shook the psychiatric testimony industry, David Faust and Jay Ziskin, after studying the issue carefully, concluded that "professionals often fail to reach reliable or valid conclusions and . . . the accuracy of their judgments does not necessarily surpass that of laypersons, thus raising substantial doubt that psychologists or psychiatrists meet legal standards for expertise." Faust and Ziskin cited as supportive research:

- A study showing that psychiatrists viewing the same psychiatric interviews could not agree on patients' diagnoses, motivations, or conscious and unconscious feelings.
- A study of military recruits who were retained despite psychiatrists' recommendations that they be discharged for mental instability. "After two years," Faust and Ziskin note, "most of these individuals had remained on active duty and their overall rate of success and adjustment was not substantially different from that of matched controls initially judged to be free of pathology."
- A study showing that psychiatrists who interviewed subjects were no better at obtaining information about their mental states than lay interviewers using standardized forms.

In short, psychiatrists and psychologists are no better at understanding people's past and present mental states, or predicting their future behavior, than you are—and they have no right to make such predictions in court cases when people's lives are at stake. As Faust and Ziskin point out, psychiatric and psychological expert witnesses fail to meet the two legal standards for expertise: (1) the ability to achieve reasonable certainty about the issues they're testifying on, and (2) the ability to help the judge and jury reach a more accurate decision than would otherwise be possible. When it comes to decisions regarding future behavior of criminals,

Faust and Ziskin are even more blunt: "Each time an expert witness claims he can predict violent behavior with reasonable certainty, he endorses a falsehood." (This is fairly mild compared to the reaction of one former head of the American Psychiatric Association, who labeled psychiatric expert witnesses who make such predictions as "a bunch of clowns.")

The only legitimate role a psychiatrist can play in a courtroom is as a medical doctor, testifying about the presence or absence of scientifically verifiable disorders. A psychiatrist can testify with a clear conscience as to whether a criminal has Wilson's disease, a thyroid disorder, a brain tumor, or any other disorder that can be verified by a careful evaluation. The psychiatrist can even make some tentative assumptions about whether a defendant's behavior may have been influenced by such physical disorders. Beyond that, however, a psychiatrist has no business testifying about a defendant's mental state at the time a crime was committed, or about his or her likelihood of committing future crimes—especially if such guesses are based on meaningless DSM labels.

"An expert in a courtroom setting is supposed to be competent to present an opinion with reasonable certainty," researcher Robyn Dawes says, in *House of Cards*. "But a mental health expert who expresses a confident opinion about the probable future behavior of a single individual . . . is by definition incompetent, because the research has demonstrated that neither a mental health expert nor anyone else can make such a prediction with accuracy sufficient to warrant much confidence."

The poor record of psychological and psychiatric expert witnesses is not surprising. After all, most "experts" base their testimony on DSM—and DSM labels are subjective, unscientific, and so broadly written that they can be stretched to fit any conclusion a psychiatrist or psychologist is expected to reach. (That's why we so often hear of trials in which the defendant is labeled by three different doctors as having three entirely different conditions.) Few psychiatrists physically examine the subjects they're testifying for or against, and of course no psychologists do. Given that even a skilled physician who knows the correct diagnosis of a patient's brain dysfunction can't always predict what the patient will do as a result of the dysfunction, predictions based on a system of simplistic and inaccurate labels are bound to be wrong as often as they're right. The "diagnoses" and predictions of psychoanalytically oriented psychiatrists, in particular, often appear to be based on conclusions drawn out of thin air.

Good examples of this can be found in *Alone With the Devil*, by Ronald Markman, M.D. Markman, a forensic psychiatrist in Los Angeles, specializes in determining the "mental states" of criminals, and has interviewed everyone from members of Charles Manson's "family" to Juan Corona and the Hillside Strangler, Kenneth Bianchi. Markman has played a role in dozens of criminal cases in California over the past few decades. He has been asked to decide whether movie director Roman Polanski was a mentally disordered sex offender, whether Manson family member Leslie Van Houten should stand trail for murder, and whether Richard Chase—the "Vampire of Sacramento"—was crazy. How did Markman come to his conclusions? "I guess you could say my goal is to get inside the mind of the killer," he says, in *Alone With the Devil*. "I do this by interviewing the person, usually across a small table, alone."

Interviewing a person across a small table may indeed yield some clues as to whether he or she is "insane"—but it certainly won't tell you why. To Markman's credit, he appears to have referred some of his interviewees to other doctors for physical exams, when the symptoms of their medical disorders (tumors, and so on) were fairly obvious. But Markman seems not to have conducted thorough neuromedical evaluations of his subjects himself. Thus, I'm not surprised at some of his "diagnoses."

* * *

Markman was involved in the trial of Orlando Camacho, who brutally murdered his wife because he was obsessed with the idea (which was untrue) that she was having sex with many men while he was gone. Camacho decapitated Elizabeth Camacho, but hallucinated for days afterward that her head was still conversing with him.

Markman, asked to decide whether Camacho was fit to stand trial, concluded that the man was psychotic. (A fairly simple "diagnosis" to make, when your patient decapitates his wife and carries on conversations with her head!) But *why* did Camacho snap? Without examining Camacho, I wouldn't have a clue. He might have had a tumor, or a disorder that causes temporal lobe seizures. He might have suffered from chronic insecticide poisoning, drug-induced brain dysfunction, encephalitis, or any number of other disorders.

Markman, however, doesn't mention investigating any of these possibilities. To him, Camacho's problem was clear. Noting that the man had shown no evidence of insane behavior until shortly before murdering his wife, Markman said, "There always has to be a first time [for a psychotic episode]—and it's usually associated with a definable, specific stress. You can always find it if you look long and hard enough." And what stress did Markman identify? Camacho's recent marriage to Elizabeth. "Marriage is a stress in anyone's life," he says. Well, yes. But ask yourself: of all the married men you've known during your life, how many were driven by the stress of saying "I do" to break candlesticks over their wives' heads, attempt to suffocate them with pillows, and then decapitate them with butter knives?

* * *

Another case in which Markman participated involved a young man who murdered his infant son. The man, a fourth-year seminary student in the Mormon Church, appeared to be the ideal husband and father. By all accounts, he doted on his wife, loved his son, and was a wonderful undergraduate teacher and devoted church member. He apparently had no history of bizarre or even unlikable behavior, except for some odd feelings during his migraine headaches.

Shortly before the murder, his headaches became savage. Although he had suffered a few such headaches previously, the ones he experienced in the weeks before killing his son apparently were unbearable. He visited a chiropractor, and was told that the headaches were due to low blood sugar and a displaced vertebra in his neck. Most likely, however, they were due to a much more serious brain dysfunction—one that probably led to the bizarre hallucinations he began having shortly afterward. During one of these hallucinations, the man became convinced that God was calling on him to sacrifice his son as Abraham had been asked to sacrifice Isaac. He stabbed the baby with a kitchen knife.

What did Markman have to say about this? He agreed with the physicians at Utah State Hospital, who concluded that the man had suffered from "atypical psychosis." Why? Because "following what he believed to be the strictures and requirements of his religious faith, he cultivated powerful frustrations and resentments. Yet he could neither acknowledge nor express them." Thus, Markman concluded, the man was forced to express his frustrations in a religious "drama." (Millions of people from very religious families occasionally feel restricted or frustrated by the rules their beliefs impose on them. But how many of them, in any given year, ritually slaughter their children as a result?)

Because he was labeled as being "psychotic" at the time of his crime, the man was confined to Utah State Hospital. After about three years, he was released. At the time Markman's book was published (1989), the man was living with his wife and their second child in Utah. Given that the specific cause of the brain dysfunction that caused this man to "snap" apparently was never uncovered—a label of "atypical psychosis" doesn't tell us what *caused* the psychosis—there is no way to know whether he could become violent again.

*   *   *

Thousands of similar "diagnoses" are being made every day by forensic psychiatrists. Every day, murderers and other criminals are judged as "sane" or "insane" by psychiatrists sitting across interview tables and applying DSM labels. Every day, formerly violent prisoners are released on parole because a psychiatric evaluation has stated that they are "no longer a threat"—and other convicts are sent back to jail because of reports saying that they are still dangerous. But virtually none of these decisions has any basis in medical fact.

An excellent recent example of the illogicality of much psychiatric testimony was the trial of Jeffrey Dahmer, the Milwaukee man who murdered at least 17 young men (apparently in an attempt to turn them into "zombies") and ate parts of their bodies. The psychiatrists asked to testify about what ailed Dahmer offered up a plethora of DSM labels: paraphilia, "personality disorder not otherwise specified," antisocial personality disorder, obsessive-compulsive behavior, even "sexual disorder not otherwise specified." Based on these strange and conflicting "diagnoses," the psychiatrists offered their insights as to the inner workings of Dahmer's mind. One psychiatrist said Dahmer was delusional; another said his behavior was "unusual but not delusional." One said his habit of collecting victims' heads and genitals was "psychotic"; another said it was bizarre but no different than the behavior of hunters who collect animals' skins as trophies. One psychiatrist even testified that Dahmer's ability to delay gratification by putting on a condom before having sex with his victims showed that he could conform his behavior to societal norms! Psychologist Joan Ullman, reporting on the trial in *Psychology Today,* summed up the psychiatric testimony as "crazy-sounding arguments pushed to logical absurdities by expert witnesses you could only regard as hired goons."

Despite the obvious silliness of such testimony, psychiatrists and psychologists continue to wield considerable power in the courtroom, often with far-reaching effects on our personal liberties. One reason is that courts have historically required, when considering whether an individual qualifies as an expert witness, that the witness's beliefs or methods be "generally accepted" within his or her field. Unfortunately, psychologists and psychiatrists using

DSM labels are indeed practicing state-of-the-art methods, according to their respective professional groups. And even when psychiatric and psychological testimony can be shown to be no better than guesswork, it is still generally accepted. The U.S. Supreme Court acknowledged, in 1983, that psychiatrists' predictions of future dangerous behavior by patients were wrong twice as often as they were right, but still allowed such testimony. "Neither [party in the case] suggests that psychiatrists are always wrong with respect to future dangerousness, only most of the time," the Court said in an odd ruling.

Unfortunately, psychiatric witnesses who are wrong "most of the time" can cause a great deal of harm. We're all familiar with cases in which criminals labeled as "rehabilitated" by psychiatrists have been released, only to kill or rape again within hours. One five-year study of defendants judged not guilty by reason of insanity, and then released to community programs when their doctors said they were "no longer a danger to society," found that one-third had been arrested again—mostly for violent offenses. Conversely, psychiatric testimony wrongly labels many defendants as a threat to society. In one study, cited by Faust and Ziskin, researchers tracked 967 people whom psychiatrists had labeled as violent and dangerous; four years after they had received these labels, only 26 of these individuals had committed violent or dangerous acts.

But if psychiatrists aren't good at judging convicted criminals' future actions, they're certainly good at keeping lawbreakers out of jail in the first place. The DSM "diagnosis" is an invaluable tool in this effort, because virtually anyone can qualify as disabled by DSM standards and, thus, is not responsible for his or her actions. Here are some examples of how psychiatrists testifying for defendants have used the flexibility of DSM to the defendants' advantage:

- In 1985, Lisa Grimshaw, her boyfriend, and another man drive to a boat ramp where she dropped the men off—along with two baseball bats. Then Lisa picked up her estranged husband at his workplace and drove him to the boat ramp, proposing a romantic interlude. When he left the car, the two men jumped out from hiding and beat him to death with the bats. Despite her participation in this cold-blooded murder, Lisa got off on a reduced charge—manslaughter—because her lawyer was able to find a doctor who testified that she suffered from posttraumatic stress disorder (PTSD).

- Michael Tindall was caught flying drugs into the United States. He was acquitted when an expert witness convinced the jury that he was suffering from posttraumatic stress disorder as a result of a tour of duty in Vietnam. Another veteran was acquitted of attempting to kill his ex-wife after experts told jurors he was suffering from PTSD.

Posttraumatic stress disorder is the most successful method of convincing jurors that defendants are "psychiatrically disturbed," and therefore not accountable for their acts, but DSM is full of similarly useful labels. ("Multiple personality disorder," for example, allows defendants to claim that "other personalities" committed acts without their knowledge.) Furthermore, the number of DSM "it's-not-my-fault" excuses for murder and mayhem is likely to grow rather than diminish in the future, because both psychiatrists and lawyers are already pushing for additional labels. Granted, some proposed dream defenses have been kept out: "sadistic personality disorder," which could be used to excuse many cases of spouse battering, was included in DSM-III-R but removed from DSM-IV; and "paraphiliac coercive disorder," which would label men who become aroused by committing violent acts as "disabled," was voted down. But attorneys and other interest groups are lobbying strongly for these "diagnoses":

- "Victimization disorder," in which people who have been victimized themselves feel compelled to victimize others.
- "Oppression artifact disorder," which would excuse criminal or violent behavior on the basis that it was committed by a member of a frequently oppressed minority group.

"These aspiring disorders can be expected to receive powerful lobbying support," Nancy Watzman and William Saletan warn, in *The New Republic*. "Together, the mental health professionals who define new diseases and the lawyers who labor to broaden their definitions form an emerging industry that recasts people's unfortunate life histories as the root causes of ailments, which can . . . insulate them from criminal responsibility."

This industry is a very profitable one: some "professional experts" pull in as much as $200,000 a year in extra income. Needless to say, a system in which psychiatrists and psychologists in effect get paid to apply DSM labels favorable to one client or another is an invitation to questionable practices by practitioners looking for additional income. One sign of ethical degradation is the growing number of "witness brokers" willing to find a psychiatrist or psychologist who is a "good match" for an attorney—a polite way of saying a hired gun who is virtually guaranteed to say what the lawyer wants. Although these experts don't get paid more when clients win than when they lose, it's tacitly accepted that those who help obtain judgments favorable to their clients will get more referrals in the future.

As psychiatrist Thomas Szasz has put it succinctly, in criminal trials "there are two types of psychiatrists: excusers and incriminators. The former, hired by the defense, are paid to offer psychiatric prevarications that tend to excuse the accused. The latter, hired by the prosecution, are paid to offer psychiatric prevarications tending to incriminate the accused. If a psychiatrist is unwilling to offer such testimony, he is not hired." And a psychiatrist who does have the courage to testify honestly on the stand, even if it hurts the hiring lawyer's case, isn't likely to be hired a second time.

This abuse of the legal system by psychiatric expert witnesses ensures further weakening of psychiatry's poor reputation as a science and a field of medicine. "As the courts and the public come to realize the immense gap between experts' claims about their judgmental powers and the scientific findings," Faust and Ziskin predict, "the credibility of psychology and psychiatry will suffer accordingly." But perhaps that suffering will be all for the good: it may teach us to be more cautious about putting so much power in the hands of "experts" armed with nothing more than a book of empty labels.

What psychiatrists are doing in America's courtrooms is often, in my opinion, unconscionable. But the true tragedy of psychiatry's abuse of the justice system is that there *is* a valid role for psychiatrists in the criminal justice system—a role that psychiatrists are not performing. That role consists of identifying and, when possible, correcting, the brain disorders of criminal offenders. There's strong evidence that a significant percentage of hard-core criminals suffer from serious brain dysfunctions—and that society could be saved much grief and expense if psychiatry focused on understanding the causes and aiding in the treatment or prevention of such disfunctions. For example:

- H. G. Brunner and colleagues have strongly linked a genetic defect to violent behavior in some males. Studying a large family tree, the researchers found that all of the male members with the defective gene were mildly mentally retarded and had a history of reacting aggressively and impulsively when challenged. Crimes committed by the affected males included arson, attempted rape, and exhibitionism.
- A recent study by Deborah Denno found that high lead levels were the strongest predictor of behavior problems in school—which, in turn, were the strongest predictor of delinquency. Other studies have linked high lead levels to hyperactivity, attention deficit, reduced IQ, and poor frustration tolerance—all of which are major risk factors for criminal behavior.
- One study found that, of 31 men who violently abused their wives, 19 had a history of severe head injury; this, researchers Alan Rosenbaum and Steven Hoge noted, is "61 percent, a proportion far greater than the rate of head injury

in the general population, estimated at around six percent." Another study by Rosenbaum and colleagues, of wife-beaters and two control groups (happily and unhappily married men who did not abuse their wives), found that "a history of significant head injury increased the chances of marital aggression almost six-fold."

- Abnormally low levels of the brain chemical serotonin are strongly linked to aggression, suicide, and impulsive psychopathic crimes. And low serotonin levels, in turn, are caused by a variety of underlying brain dysfunction—none of which is cured by doctors who simply administer Prozac to artificially adjust serotonin levels, without addressing the issue of why serotonin levels were abnormal in the first place.

- Researchers V. H. Mark and F. R. Ervin have studied a behavior pattern they call "dyscontrol syndrome," consisting of physical assaults on others; an odd reaction to alcohol, in which even light drinking triggers acts of senseless violence; a history of impulsive sexual behavior, sometimes including assault or rape; and a history of serious traffic violations and car accidents. Studying 400 prisoners with this behavior pattern, they found strong evidence linking symptoms of "dyscontrol" to brain dysfunction, evidenced in seizures and other abnormalities.

All in all, dozens of medical conditions or diseases can cause or contribute to violent or criminal behavior. They range from liver and kidney disease to Cushing's disease, thyroid disorders, lupus, heavy-metal poisoning, and porphyria. And many of these conditions can be diagnosed and corrected.

It would be simplistic to blame all crime on brain dysfunction. And many biological causes of crime, even when they can be diagnosed, can't yet be corrected. Our risk of being victims of crime could be substantially reduced, however, if those biologically at risk for criminal behavior could be diagnosed early—or, at worst, following their first few offenses—and, when possible, could receive treatment to correct their brain dysfunctions.

Yet, tragically, studies show that almost no criminal offenders receive thorough medical examinations. By abdicating their role in diagnosing and treating brain dysfunctions that can lead to continued criminal behavior, and choosing instead to grandstand in the courtrooms, psychiatrists working in America's judicial system are endangering all of us.

Getting DSM Out of Our Lives

Unfortunately, there's not much advice I can give nonpatients about how to avoid being "DSMed." The manual has become such a pervasive part of our legal system and our society in general that anyone is at risk. There's not much you can do, for instance, to stop your ex-wife or ex-husband from finding a psychiatrist who'll testify that you're "histrionic" or "adjustment disordered" and shouldn't have custody of your children. There's not much you can do to get out of hiring a kleptomaniac who's legally protected by virtue of his DSM "disability." And there's nothing you can do to stop a psychiatric expert witness from labeling a criminal who's assaulted you as "disabled" according to DSM criteria. Such abuses of psychiatry will continue, I believe, until the public and psychiatry itself see that DSM labels are not only useless as medical "diagnoses" but also have the potential to do great harm—particularly when they are used as means to deny individual freedoms, or as weapons by psychiatrists acting as hired guns for the legal system.

CHAPTER 9

Where Do We Go from Here?

Beyond Cookbook Psychiatry

Psychiatry is an emperor standing naked in his new clothes. It has worked and striven for 70 years to become an emperor, a full brother with the other medical specialties. And now it stands there resplendent in its finery. But it does not have any clothes on; and even worse, nobody has told it so.

E. Fuller Torrey,
in *The Death of Psychiatry*

MANY PEOPLE COME TO MY OFFICE AFTER SUFFERING FOR years from terrifying symptoms that have ruined their marriages, cost them their jobs, driven away their friends, or led them to attempt suicide. When I tell them what's wrong with them—and, often, tell them that it can be effectively treated or even cured—their response, almost invariably, is, "Why didn't my other psychiatrists know that?"

Why, indeed?

Most psychiatrists are dedicated doctors who truly want to help their patients. Because of their faulty training, however, many simply don't know how. I lay the blame for this squarely on the doorstep of the American Psychiatric Association, which, by publishing the DSM and holding it up as the standard for psychiatric care, has replaced diagnosis with labeling.

Modern psychiatry is, to borrow Torrey's metaphor, an emperor with no clothes, wrapped in the empty words of a "diagnostic" manual that doesn't tell doctors how to diagnose. And *you can't treat until you know what you're treating.* Until psychiatry discards the DSM method and trains its practitioners to provide real diagnosis followed by real medical management, millions of patients will be misdiagnosed, undiagnosed, and mistreated—and those lucky enough to eventually receive a diagnosis will continue to ask, "Why did I have to wait so long?"

Fortunately, the failings of DSM psychiatry are becoming increasingly apparent to its practitioners. Many psychiatrists I speak with are beginning to realize, although often only vaguely, that DSM labels, drugs, and endless psychotherapy aren't curing their patients. A number of psychiatrists are beginning to sense that the years they spent in medical school are being wasted by a system that discourages them from using their diagnostic skills. These psychiatrists know that DSM isn't working, and some of them are starting to search for an alternative.

Luckily, there *is* an alternative to DSM psychiatry. It will require good training and hard work on the part of psychiatrists, and doctors who decide to take this route will probably make less money than they're making now. They'll have problems dealing with insurance companies, other psychiatrists, and mental health care facilities. And they'll probably lose a few patients who are seeking a quick Prozac "cure." What they'll gain, in return, is the very thing most of them went into medicine to achieve: the satisfaction of helping patients by diagnosing and treating disease. I'm optimistic enough to be convinced that, for most psychiatrists, this satisfaction will more than compensate for the bureaucratic hassles they will encounter.

The alternative I'm proposing is the science of *deductive differential diagnosis.* It's time for psychiatrists to return to being physicians—not seers, priests, gurus, or pill pushers, but real physicians. It's time for them to start asking what's *really* wrong with their "hyperactive," "depressed," and "anxious" patients, and to start uncovering and treating the causes of their problems—not just hiding their symptoms under layers of dangerous and addictive drugs. And, above all, it's time for psychiatrists to abandon the flaky idea that they are treating an invisible "mind," and realize that all of the emotional, behavioral, and thought problems they treat stem from disordered brain cells (neurons).

This realization, in my opinion, is the key to the future of psychiatry. In fact, I believe an entirely new approach to psychiatry— *clinical neuronal reductivism*—should replace the DSM. The term, admittedly a mouthful, simply means that disorders must be traced, whenever possible, to malfunctions in the brain cells themselves, and to abnormalities in the chemical "soup" in which they live. As the late, great Dr. Derek Denny-Brown, Putnam Professor of Neurology at Harvard Medical School, once put it, "to better understand behavior one must characterize the environment of the neuron."

This means, in plain English, looking beyond labels such as "depression" and "anxiety," and seeking the *causes* of despondency, anxiety, and hopelessness. It means determining and treating these causes, rather than masking them with drugs. It means ceasing to blame mothers, fathers, schools, or society for problems stemming from malfunctioning brain cells. And it means directing research toward finding cures for the disorders that ail these malfunctioning cells, rather than simply making up new names for them.

Advances in medical science—from gene mapping to brain scanning—have given us an opportunity, unknown to the physicians who came before us, to understand the workings of the brain and its cells. If we accept the challenge of practicing 21st-century medicine, and use the medical tools and knowledge available to us to treat brain disorders, our patients and the field of psychiatry itself will benefit. Should we choose to stagnate, and continue to label and drug and psychoanalyze patients rather than diagnosing and treating them, psychiatry may die an iatrogenic death—killed by its own hand. The choice is ours.

Taking a Stand

If sweeping changes are to occur in psychiatry, they will require a moral as well as a scientific revolution. To accomplish it, psychiatrists will need to take a strong stand against the overdrugging, nondiagnosis, and nontreatment of psychiatric patients—and the drugging and overtreatment of patients who have no disorders at all.

Admittedly, taking this stand will require courage, because the special interests involved in maintaining psychiatry's status quo are huge and astonishingly powerful. Psychiatrists attempting to change the DSM system must be prepared to meet them head-on.

THE DRUG COMPANIES

Drug company money influences every aspect of modern-day psychiatry. The American Psychiatric Association is literally built on a foundation of drug money: millions of dollars of pharmaceutical advertising money are poured into the APA's publications, conferences, continuing education programs, and seminars. In return, the APA bends over backward to help drug companies promote their products. (A typical example of this incestuous relationship, cited in *Consumer Reports,* was a seminar, at the 1991 annual meeting of the American Psychiatric Association, that focused on the treatment of manic depression. "Despite the broad topic," the magazine reported, "the session mainly focused on the use of anticonvulsant drugs, even though the FDA has never approved them for this use." Why? Because the symposium was sponsored by the company that sold Depakote, an anticonvulsant drug.) And 15 to 20 percent of the APA's income in recent years has come directly from drug company advertising in APA journals—another means of guaranteeing good press for new drugs.

Given that the APA owes much of its financial stability to the drug companies, it isn't likely to challenge any of these questionable practices. When several members of the APA board of trustees once questioned the pervasive influence of drug money on the organization, the APA responded by forming a Task Force to Study the Impact of the Potential Loss of Pharmaceutical Support—a revealing title—which concluded, in effect, that the APA couldn't continue to function without massive drug industry subsidies. So ethical concerns were cast aside, and drug companies have continued to exercise considerable (although unofficial) influence over the APA.

That influence, to a large degree, has focused on expanding the number of "psychiatric disorders" recognized by the APA, and the number of drug treatments recommended for these disorders. After all, every DSM "diagnosis" is a potential gold mine for pharmaceutical firms. For instance, before PMS was listed as a "psychiatric disorder," most doctors might have hesitated to prescribe powerful and potentially dangerous psychiatric drugs for moderate PMS symptoms. Most would probably have advised their patients to eat right, cut down on caffeine and sugar, exercise, or take a few aspirin. And most would have assumed that severe PMS, being a physical disorder, would indicate the need for good endocrine and OB/GYN workups. But now PMS is officially enshrined as a "mental" disorder in the DSM (under "premenstrual dysphoric disorder"). It's only in the appendix of DSM-IV at the moment, but a number of psychiatrists are lobbying to have it declared a full-fledged diagnosis. If and when that happens, the drug companies stand to profit handsomely. Why? Because, under DSM criteria, as many as half a million American women will be thought of as "disabled" once a month. And "disabled" women, according to current psychiatric thinking, need prescriptions. (Already, doctors are pushing antidepressants as a "treatment" for PMS.)

It's no surprise, therefore, that drug companies were among those encouraging the APA to include PMS in the manual. And it's no surprise that drug companies are funding much of the research into PMS and drug "treatments" for the condition.

In a similar fashion, pharmaceutical companies have supported DSM's "bracket creep," which increasingly defines perfectly healthy people as disabled. Over the past few decades, millions of Americans once thought of as normal have been labeled by DSM as having "disorders"—shyness, histrionic personality, dependency—requiring medical intervention. (Even "chocoholism," a strong craving for chocolate, is now being considered a "compulsive" disorder and is being treated with injections of the drug naloxone.) Each time DSM broadens the definition of abnormality, a new market for psychotropic drugs opens up. An expanded market translates, of course, into millions of dollars of additional profits for drug companies.

So be prepared for drug companies to exert their considerable powers to keep the DSM, and its ever-expanding list of "diagnoses," as the status quo for psychiatry. They'll oppose any efforts to replace the current label-and-drug system of psychiatry with diagnostic methods that would drastically cut the amounts of psychotropic drugs prescribed. How can they do this? By using their tremendous financial clout to influence the APA, its members, and the general public. By throwing research money in the direction of psychiatrists who support DSM-and-drug psychiatry, and refusing to fund research that might reduce the use of drugs in the treatment of psychiatric patients. And by massaging the results of the research they fund in order to "prove," in virtually every case, the existence of new "psychiatric disorders" and the need to treat them with new drugs.

THE AMERICAN PSYCHIATRIC ASSOCIATION (APA)

The APA is a mighty force, with more than 35,000 members, a staff of lobbyists, and a hefty annual income (much of it, as I've noted, from drug companies). And the APA doesn't hesitate to use these resources to put pressure on maverick psychiatrists; just ask Thomas Szasz and E. Fuller Torrey, who were punished severely for taking on the APA. Szasz, the first major psychiatrist to question the labeling of psychiatric patients, said in *Society* that "by 1970, I had become a non-person in American psychiatry. The pages of American psychiatric journals were shut to my work. Soon, the very mention of my name became taboo and was omitted from new editions of texts that had previously featured my views. In short, I became the object of that most effective of all criticisms, the silent treatment." As for Torrey, a pioneering psychiatrist who was among the first to insist that schizophrenia was a biological disorder, he was booted out of the American Psychiatric Association altogether.

Although such extreme reactions by the APA are rare, questioning this powerful organization can be dangerous to a psychiatrist's professional health. Being "in" with the APA can help a psychiatrist gain prestige, publish in important journals, get speaking engagements at conferences, and obtain lucrative teaching or research positions. Conversely, doctors who challenge the APA's dogma can find themselves unofficially blackballed. They may discover that they aren't being invited to present papers at seminars or to publish articles in APA journals. And they may find it increasingly hard to obtain positions at universities or hospitals.

But, you may ask, won't the APA look favorably on improvements to a "diagnostic" system it must know is riddled with nonscience and politics? Not likely. The history of the APA has been one of ruthless opposition to any proposed changes to its status quo. This attitude, I hasten to add, exists not just within the APA, but in just about every field of medicine. (Australian doctors Barry Marshall and J. Robin Warren, for instance, spent years trying to convince other doctors that many ulcers were caused by simple bacteria that could be killed with antibiotics. For their troubles, they were exiled from professional meetings, ignored by most medical journals, and either laughed at or shunned by their colleagues. Turns out that they were right all along—but it took 11 years for the medical community to admit it.) But although all fields of medicine are obstinate about accepting change, the field of psychiatry is the most closed-minded. That's because other medical fields are based on science and hard evidence, and even the most stubborn doctors, presented with enough evidence, will eventually change their minds. Psychiatry, unfortunately, has always been based more on subjective philosophy than on scientific facts—so all of the evidence in the world isn't likely to persuade it to change its course.

HMOs, Psychiatric Hospitals, and Insurance Companies

Careful diagnostic procedures, as I've mentioned earlier, are often frowned on by HMOs and psychiatric hospitals, which want maximum profit at minimal cost. Psychiatrists who put their patients' interests first aren't likely to survive in these programs, which usually insist on rapid patient turnaround, DSM labels, and only enough tests to cover their liability. "It used to be that the good doctor was the old-fashioned careful guy who ran all the tests and took care of his patients," says physician Sanford Marcus, a critic of the HMO movement. "That's a bad doctor now. The good one is the one who can bring in a lot of short-turnover, easy-care patients." A "good" psychiatrist, according to the new philosophy, is one who can choose a DSM label, write a prescription, and have a patient out the door in 15 minutes or less. A "bad" psychiatrist, conversely, is one who actually diagnoses and treats patients. Thus, psychiatrists who forgo DSM labels and offer their patients real diagnoses and treatments may find it difficult or impossible to function within the setting of an HMO or for-profit hospital.

They may, in addition, find it difficult to obtain reimbursement from insurance companies. Insurers like DSM "diagnoses," because they think they're cheap. Why? First of all, many policies pay far less for "psychiatric" illnesses than for "real" illnesses—usually 50 percent as opposed to 80 percent. Thus, a patient labeled as "depressed" gets reimbursed a great deal less than a patient who's diagnosed as having a thyroid disorder or infection. Furthermore, because a DSM label can be applied right in the office, after a minimal evaluation, and with no need for outside evaluations, referrals, or tests, the typical DSM diagnosis looks like a real bargain from an insurance company's point of view.

It isn't a bargain at all. For years, I've tried to convince insurers that it makes sense to spend an extra few hundred dollars up front for a real diagnosis and treatment. After all, tumors, thyroid disorders, infections, and other medical problems don't go away when a DSM label is applied; they simply cause more serious and more expensive problems in the future. Furthermore, it makes more sense to diagnose and treat patients up front than to put them on costly medications that often make them sicker.

Unfortunately, most insurance companies think in the short term. It really doesn't matter to them whether a patient with a slow-growing tumor rings up a huge hospital bill ten years from now, as long as that patient gets treated "on the cheap" now. Thus, doctors opting to diagnose and treat patients, and refusing to simply label them, are likely to spend a good part of their time fighting with insurers more concerned about DSM codes than about patient welfare.

A Worthwhile Risk

In short, psychiatrists who take on the DSM myth may find themselves doing battle with powerful opponents, some of whom will stop at little to silence them. I know this from firsthand experience, and I'm not issuing my challenge to the timid. I'm aware that psychiatrists who throw out their DSMs will face formidable obstacles. But in every revolution, the leaders take risks—and what I'm recommending is indeed a revolution in the medical care of patients with brain dysfunctions. It won't be a small revolution, either, but one in which the lives and health of millions of patients are at stake.

Doctors who join this revolution won't be the first to challenge the psychiatric establishment. Only a few decades ago, autistic patients were being psychoanalyzed, schizophrenic patients were being lobotomized, and patients with the nutritional disorder pellagra were being confined to mental institutions for life. The doctors who challenged those treatments were ostracized, but in the long run they prevailed. It's not easy to change psychiatry—but it's not impossible, either. We owe it to ourselves, and to our patients, to try.

How Patients Can Help

What can you, as a consumer of psychiatric services, do to participate in this revolution?

First, and most important, change the way you deal with psychiatrists. Refuse to pay huge sums for psychiatric "treatments" that don't work. Refuse to let a psychiatrist prescribe Ritalin for your "hyperactive" child's symptoms, without even performing an examination. Refuse to accept a prescription for your "anxiety" or "depression" from a doctor who has spent only 15 minutes evaluating you. Insist on a real diagnosis, and walk away from any psychiatrist who won't provide one.

Second, refuse to fall for the seductive message that psychiatric drugs can cushion life's blows or make you a better person. Say no if a psychiatrist suggests that taking Prozac will make you more confident, more energetic, or more attractive. Refuse to escape from stresses and life traumas by taking Valium, Xanax, and other potentially addictive drugs.

What else? Avoid codependency therapies, repressed memory therapies, and other dangerous "pop-psych" techniques that have no basis in science or reason. Accept responsibility for your own health and keep your body, and your brain, in good shape, by eating right, exercising, sleeping well, and following common-sense health rules. If something goes wrong anyway, spend the time and money necessary to find a good physician who will uncover your problems instead of hiding them with drugs.

Above all, be a skeptic. Listen to your doctors, but don't assume that they're always right. Ask them why they prescribe drugs or other treatments. Look up the benefits and risks of treatments yourself, rather than relying solely on your doctors' recommendations. Get second opinions when major decisions are involved. Become the kind of patient many psychiatrists dread: a fully informed, confident, and assertive participant in your own health care decisions. For too long, American medicine—and psychiatry in particular—has treated its patients as passive, ignorant, trusting dependents. Break that habit, and insist on being a full partner in your medical care.

I hope that, after reading this book, you'll want to take that responsibility. And I hope you'll take away the message that psychiatry gone wrong has the potential to damage or even destroy you—while psychiatry at its best has tremendous potential to save your sanity and your life. It can't do either, however, without your cooperation.

References

Chapter 1 Typhus, Tattoos, and Waterbeds

1 Gray, Melvin, *Neuroses: A Comprehensive and Critical View.* New York: Van Nostrand Reinhold Co., 1978.

1 Caplan, Paula J., *They Say You're Crazy.* Reading, MA: Addison-Wesley Publishing Co., 1995.

5 Dumont, Matthew P., "A diagnostic parable (first edition—unrevised)," *Readings: A Journal of Reviews and Commentary in Mental Health,* Vol. 2, No. 4, December 1987.

5 Taylor, Robert L., *Mind or Body: Distinguishing Psychological from Organic Disorders.* New York: McGraw-Hill, 1982.

5 *Diagnostic and Statistical Manual of Mental Disorders,* Fourth Edition. Washington, DC: American Psychiatric Press, 1994.

7 Dawes, Robyn, *House of Cards: Psychology and Psychotherapy Built on Myth.* New York: The Free Press, 1994.

13 Hoffman, Robert, study cited in *Science News,* Vol. 122, September 11, 1982.

13 Herring, M. M., "Debate over 'false-positive schizophrenics,'" *Medicine Tribune,* September 25, 1985, page 3.

13 Koranyi, Erwin K., "Undiagnosed physical illness in psychiatric patients," *Annual Review of Medicine,* Vol. 33, 1982.

14 Koran, Lorrin, study cited in "Medical evaluation of psychiatric patients," *American Family Physician,* Vol. 41, No. 4, April 1990.

14   Inlander, Charles B., Levin, Lowell S., and Weiner, Ed, *Medicine on Trial*. Englewood Cliffs, NJ: Prentice-Hall Press, 1988.

14   Walshe, Sir Francis, cited in Sydney Walker III, *Psychiatric Signs and Symptoms Due to Medical Problems*. New York: Charles C. Thomas, 1967.

16   Torrey, E. Fuller, *The Mind Game: Witchdoctors and Psychiatrists* (revised edition). New York: Harper & Row, 1986.

16   Carstairs, G. M., observations cited in E. Fuller Torrey, *The Mind Game* (*id.*).

16   Allen, Frances, cited in Ann Japenga, "Rewriting the dictionary of madness," *Los Angeles Times Magazine*, June 5, 1994.

18   Maxmen, Jerrold, *The New Psychiatry*. New York: William Morrow and Co., 1985.

20   Armstrong, Louise, *And They Call It Help*. Reading, MA: Addison-Wesley Publishing Co., 1993.

21   Kirk, Stuart A., and Kutchins, Herb, *The Selling of DSM: The Rhetoric of Science in Psychiatry*. New York: Aldine de Gruyter, 1992.

21   Matulis, Jean, cited in Ann Japenga, "Rewriting the dictionary of madness," *Los Angeles Times Magazine*, June 5, 1994.

22   Garfinkel, Renee, cited in Paula J. Caplan, *They Say You're Crazy*. Reading, MA: Addison-Wesley Publishing Co., 1995.

22   Masson, Jeffrey Moussaieff, *Final Analysis: The Making and Unmaking of a Psychoanalyst*. Reading, MA: Addison-Wesley Publishing Co., 1990.

Chapter 2   The Psychiatric Bible and the Dangers of Misdiagnosis

27   Fabricant, Noah, cited in Colin Jarman, *The Guinness Book of Poisonous Quotes*. Chicago: Contemporary Books, 1993.

27   Skrabanek, Petr, and McCormick, James, *Follies and Fallacies in Medicine*. Buffalo: Prometheus Books, 1990.

29   Spitzer, Robert, et al., *DSM-IV Casebook*. Washington, DC: American Psychiatric Press, 1994.

31   Torrey, E. Fuller, *The Death of Psychiatry*. Radnor, PA: Chilton Book Co., 1974.

31   Rimland, Bernard, "Plain talk about PDD and the diagnosis of autism," *Autism Research Review International*, Vol. 7, No. 2, 1993.

32   *Diagnostic and Statistical Manual of Mental Disorders,* Fourth Edition. Washington, DC: American Psychiatric Press, 1994.

38   Caplan, Paula J., *They Say You're Crazy.* Reading, MA: Addison-Wesley Publishing Co., 1995.

39   Brewer, George J., and Yuzbasiyan-Gurkan, Vilma, "Wilson disease," *Medicine,* Vol. 71, No. 3, May 1992.

44   Kra, Siegfried, *Aging Myths: Reversible Causes of Mind and Memory Loss.* New York: McGraw-Hill Book Co., 1986.

47   Maxmen, Jerrold, *The New Psychiatry.* New York: William Morrow and Co., 1985.

50   Dumont, Matthew P., "A diagnostic parable (first edition—unrevised)," *Readings: A Journal of Reviews and Commentary in Mental Health,* Vol. 2, No. 4, December 1987.

Chapter 3   Bad Medicine

57   Miguel, E. C., et al., "Psychiatric manifestations of systemic lupus erythematosus: clinical features, symptoms, and signs of central nervous system activity in 43 patients," *Medicine,* Vol. 73, No. 4, July 1994.

58   Twerski, Abraham, *Who Says You're Neurotic?* Englewood Cliffs, NJ: Prentice-Hall, Inc., 1984.

59   Eisenberg, Leon, cited in Antonia Black, "The drugging of America's children," *Redbook,* December 1994.

62   Boyd, Richard D., "Neuroleptic malignant syndrome and mental retardation: review and analysis of 29 cases," *American Journal on Mental Retardation,* Vol. 98, No. 1, 1993.

62   Studies in the *Journal of Clinical Psychiatry* on antidepressants and sexual dysfunction cited in Susan Brink, "Singing the Prozac blues," *U.S. News & World Report,* November 8, 1993.

63   Gladstone, Robert, and Yudofsky, Stuart, cited in "High anxiety," *Consumer Reports,* Vol. 58, No. 1, 1993.

63   Riddle, Mark, Geller, Barbara, and Ryan, Neal, "Another sudden death in a child treated with desipramine," *Journal of the American Academy of Child and Adolescent Psychiatry,* Vol. 32, No. 4, 1993.

63   Thorogood, Margaret, "Fatal myocardial infarction and use of psychotropic drugs in young women," *The Lancet,* Vol. 340, No. 8827, 1992.

63   Brandes research, cited in Jean Marx, "Do antidepressants promote tumors?" *Science,* July 3, 1992. Additional studies on

Prozac and cancer, cited in Susan Brink, "A different kind of cancer risk," *U.S. News & World Report,* January 9, 1995.

64   Hillman, Alan L., Eisenberg, John M., Pauley, Mark V., Bloom, Bernard, Glick, Henry, Kinosian, Bruce, and Schwartz, J. Sanford, "Avoiding bias in the conduct and reporting of cost-effectiveness research sponsored by pharmaceutical companies," *New England Journal of Medicine,* Vol. 324(19), May 9, 1991.

65   Upjohn-Xanax material cited in "High anxiety," *Consumer Reports,* Vol. 58, No. 1, 1993.

66   FDA investigation into Halcion, cited in Michael McCarthy, "FDA on Upjohn and Halcion," *The Lancet,* Vol. 343, No. 8907, May 14, 1994.

66   Medawar, Charles, *Power and Dependence.* London: Social Audit, Ltd., 1992.

68   *Physician's Desk Reference,* 1993.

69   Roth, Philip, cited in William Styron, "Prozac days, halcion nights: profits and pills," *The Nation,* January 4, 1993.

69   Styron, William, "Prozac days, Halcion nights: profits and pills," *The Nation,* January 4, 1993.

72   *Diagnostic and Statistical Manual of Mental Disorders,* Fourth Edition. Washington, DC: American Psychiatric Press, 1994.

74   Hughes, Richard, and Brewin, Robert, *The Tranquilizing of America.* New York: Harcourt Brace Jovanovich, 1979.

Chapter 4   Prescription Junkies

78   "High anxiety," *Consumer Reports,* Vol. 58, No. 1, January 1993.

78   Miller, Norman S., and Gold, Mark S., "Abuse, addiction, tolerance, and dependence to benzodiazepines in medical and non-medical populations," *American Journal of Drug and Alcohol Addiction,* Vol. 17, No. 1, March 1991.

78   Ricketts, Max, *The Great Anxiety Escape.* La Mesa, CA: Matulungin Publishing, 1990.

79   Bargmann, Eve, et al., *Stopping Valium.* New York: Warner Books, Inc., 1982.

79   Rickels, Karl, and Canadian Xanax studies, cited in "High anxiety," *Consumer Reports,* Vol. 58, No. 1, January 1993.

80   Zung, W. K., Daniel, J. T., King, R. E., and Moore, D. T., "A comparison of prazepam, diazepam, lorazepam and placebo in

anxious outpatients in nonpsychiatric private practices," *Journal of Clinical Psychiatry*, Vol. 42, 1989.

80   Catalan, J., Gath, D., Edmonds, G., and Ennis, J., "The effects of non-prescribing of anxiolytics in general practice—I: controlled evaluation of psychiatric and social outcome," *British Journal of Psychiatry*, Vol. 144, 1984.

80   Dilsaver, Steven, et al., "Antidepressant withdrawal syndromes: phenomenology and pathophysiology," *International Clinical Psychopharmacology*, Vol. 2, 1987.

81   Inlander, Charles B., Levin, Lowell S., and Weiner, Ed, *Medicine on Trial*. Englewood Cliffs, NJ: Hall Press, 1988.

81   Wolfe, Sidney, Fugate, Lisa, Hulstrand, Elizabeth, and Kamimoto, Laurie, *Worst Pills/Best Pills*. Washington, DC: Public Citizen Health Research Group, 1988.

81   Restak, Richard, *The Brain Has a Mind of Its Own*. New York: Harmony Books, 1991.

82   Hughes, Richard, and Brewin, Robert, *The Tranquilizing of America*. New York: Harcourt Brace Jovanovich, 1979.

83   Voth, Eric, Dupont, Robert, and Voth, Harold, "Responsible prescribing of controlled substances," *American Family Physician*, Vol. 44, No. 5, November 1991.

86   Strassman, Rick, "Hallucinogenic drugs in psychiatric research and treatment," *Journal of Nervous and Mental Disease*, Vol. 183, No. 3, 1995.

87   Kramer, Peter, *Listening to Prozac*. New York: Penguin Books, 1993.

87   Medawar, Charles, review of *Listening to Prozac*, in *Nature*, March 24, 1994.

89   Wurtzel, Elizabeth, *Prozac Nation*. Boston: Houghton Mifflin Co., 1994.

90   Safer, Daniel J., and Krager, John M., "A survey of medication treatment for hyperactive-inattentive students," *Journal of the American Medical Association*, Vol. 260, No. 15, 1988.

91   Parran, Theodore Vandoren, Jr., and Jasinski, Donald R., "Intravenous methylphenidate abuse: prototype for prescription drug abuse," *Archives of Internal Medicine*, Vol. 151, No. 4, April 1991.

91   Carter, Hayley S., and Watson, William A., "IV pentazocine/methylphenidate abuse—the clinical toxicity of another Ts and blues combination," *Journal of Toxicology*, Vol. 32, No. 5, September 1994.

91   Schmidt, Rodney A., Glenny, Robb W., Godwin, J. David, Hampson, Neil B., Cantino, Marie E., and Reichenbach,

Dennis D., "Panlobular emphysema in young intravenous Ritalin abusers," *American Review of Respiratory Diseases,* Vol. 143, No. 3, March 1991.

91 Hardman, Patricia, and Morton, Donald G., "The link between developmental dyslexia, ADD, and chemical dependency," *Environmental Medicine,* Vol. 8, No. 3, 1992.

92 Coulter, Harris L., *Vaccination, Social Violence, and Criminality.* Berkeley, CA: North Atlantic Books, 1990.

98 Quarantelli, E. L., "An assessment of conflicting views on mental health: the consequences of traumatic events," in *Trauma and its Wake, Vol. I.,* Charles R. Figley, ed. New York: Brunner/ Mazel, 1985.

100 Schnurr, Paula P., Friedman, Matthew J., and Rosenberg, Stanley D., "Premilitary MMPI scores as predictors of combat-related PTSD symptoms," *American Journal of Psychiatry,* Vol. 150, No. 3, March 1993.

102 Stevens, J., *Prescribers Journal,* 1973. Cited in Charles Medawar, *Power and Dependence.* London: Social Audit, Ltd., 1992.

Chapter 5   What's *Really* Wrong with You?

103 Rutter, Michael, "Debate and argument: There are connections between brain and mind and it is important that Rett syndrome be classified somewhere," *Journal of Child Psychology and Psychiatry,* Vol. 35, No. 2, 1994.

103 Deitrick, Frances, *I'm Not Crazy.* Far Hills, NJ: New Horizon Press, 1992.

103 Torrey, E. Fuller, *The Death of Psychiatry.* Radnor, PA: Chilton Book Co., 1974.

106 Healy, David, *The Suspended Revolution: Psychiatry and Psychotherapy Re-Examined.* London: Faber and Faber, 1990.

107 Goggans, Frederick C., Allen, Michael R., and Gold, Mark S., "Primary hypothyroidism and its relationship to affective disorders," in *Medical Mimics of Psychiatric Disorders.* Washington, DC: American Psychiatric Press, 1986.

107 Comings, David E., *Tourette Syndrome and Human Behavior.* Duarte, CA: Hope Press, 1990.

108 Dawes, Robyn, *House of Cards: Psychology and Psychotherapy Built on Myth.* New York: The Free Press, 1994.

108 Caplan, Paula J., *They Say You're Crazy*. Reading, MA: Addison-Wesley Publishing Co., 1995.

110 *Diagnostic and Statistical Manual of Mental Disorders*, Fourth Edition. Washington, DC: American Psychiatric Press, 1994.

112 Anxiety studies reported in "A false alarm: no . . . it's more Freudian," *Psychology Today*, September–October 1993.

113 Fogel, Barry S., and Slaby, Andrew E., "Neurological screening of psychiatric patients," in *Medical Mimics of Psychiatric Disorders*, Irl Extein and Mark S. Gold, eds. Washington, DC: American Psychiatric Press, 1986.

113 Klafehn, Patty Delaney, cited in Rita Baron-Faust, "Why doctors mistreat women," *Redbook*, May 1989.

114 Wassersug, Joseph D., "None of the physicians could find the coin in her throat," *American Medical News*, Vol. 34, No. 20, May 27, 1991.

114 Taylor, Robert L., *Mind or Body: Distinguishing Psychological from Organic Disorders*. New York: McGraw-Hill, 1982.

115 Tu, Jun-Bi, Shafey, Hany, and VanDewetering, Cathy, "Iron deficiency in two adolescents with conduct, dysthymic and movement disorders," *Canadian Journal of Psychiatry*, Vol. 39, August 1994.

116 Streissguth, Ann Pytkowicz, Aase, Jon M., Clarren, Sterling K., Randels, Sandra P., LaDue, Robin A., and Smith, David F., "Fetal alcohol syndrome in adolescents and adults," *Journal of the American Medical Association*, Vol. 265, No. 15, April 17, 1991.

117 Silverstein, Alvin, Silverstein, Virginia, and Silverstein, Robert, *Lyme Disease: The Great Imitator*. Lebanon, NJ: AVSTAR Publishing Corp., 1990.

117 Dobkin, Bruce, *Brain Matters*. New York: Crown Publishers, 1986.

119 Fenelon, Gilles, et al., "Munchausen's syndrome and abnormalities on magnetic resonance imaging of the brain," *British Medical Journal*, Vol. 302, No. 6783, April 27, 1991.

120 *The New Harvard Guide to Psychiatry*, Armand M. Nicholi, Jr., ed. Cambridge, MA: Belknap Press, 1988.

122 Torrey, E. Fuller, *The Death of Psychiatry*. Radnor, PA: Chilton Book Co., 1974.

123 Crick, Francis, *The Astonishing Hypothesis: The Scientific Search for the Soul*. New York: Charles Scribner's Sons, 1994.

124 Twerski, Abraham, *Who Says You're Neurotic?* Englewood Cliffs, NJ: Prentice-Hall, Inc., 1984.

124 Maxmen, Jerrold, *The New Psychiatry*. New York: William Morrow and Co., 1985.

126 Stein, D. M., and Lambert, M. J., "On the relationship between therapist experience and psychotherapy outcome," *Clinical Psychology Review*, Vol. 4, 1984.

127 Strupp, H. H., unpublished work, 1979.

127 Scogin, F., Bynum, J., Stephens, G., and Calhoon, S., "Efficacy of self-administered treatment programs: meta-analytic review," *Professional Psychology: Research and Practice*, Vol. 21, 1990.

129 Eagle, Carol, cited in Antonia Black, "The drugging of America's children," *Redbook*, December 1994.

130 Gross, Martin L., *The Psychological Society*. New York: Random House, 1978.

131 Maxmen, Jerrold, *The New Psychiatry*. New York: William Morrow and Co., 1985.

133 Caplan, Paula, J., *They Say You're Crazy*. Reading, MA: Addison-Wesley Publishing Co., 1995.

Chapter 6   Talk Soup Can Make You Sick

135 Ofshe, Richard, and Watters, Ethan, "Making monsters," *Society*, Vol. 30, No. 3, March–April 1993.

139 Breggin, Peter, *Toxic Psychiatry*. New York: St. Martin's Press, 1991.

139 Caplan, Paula J., and Hall-McCorquodale, Ian, "Mother-blaming in major clinical journals," *American Journal of Orthopsychiatry*, Vol. 55, No. 3, July 1985.

140 Frank, G. H., "The role of the family in the development of psychopathology," *Psychological Bulletin*, Vol. 64, 1965.

140 Skolnick, Arlene, "The myth of the vulnerable child," *Psychology Today*, February 1978.

140 Air Force study: Renaud, H., and Estess, F., "Life history interviews with one hundred normal American males," *American Journal of Orthopsychiatry*, Vol. 31, 1961.

141 Torrey, E. Fuller, *The Death of Psychiatry*. Radnor, PA: Chilton Book Co., 1974.

141 Macfarlane, Jean, "Perspectives on personality consistency and change from the guidance study," *Vita Humana*, Vol. 7, No. 2, 1964.

143 Breggin, Peter, and Barkley, Russell, "Q: are behavior-modifying drugs overprescribed for America's schoolchildren?," *Insight on the News,* August 14, 1995.

145 Ofshe, Richard, and Watters, Ethan, "Making monsters," *Society,* Vol. 30, No. 3, March–April 1993.

145 Pope, Harrison G., Jr., and Hudson, James I., "Can memories of childhood sexual abuse be repressed?" *Psychological Medicine,* Vol. 25, 1995.

145 Loftus, Elizabeth, and Ketcham, Katherine, *The Myth of Repressed Memory.* New York: St. Martin's Press, 1994.

146 Barden, Chris, cited in Chi Chi Sileo, "Under fire, therapy faces a backlash," *Insight on the News,* Vol. 10, No. 35, 1994.

148 Hemfelt, Robert, and Warren, Paul, *Kids Who Carry Our Pain.* Nashville: Thomas Nelson, Inc., 1990.

149 Pittman, Frank, III, "A buyer's guide to psychotherapy," *Psychology Today,* Vol. 27, No. 1, 1994.

149 Torrey, E. Fuller, "Oedipal wrecks," *The Washington Monthly,* January–February 1992.

149 Wolin, Steven, and Wolin, Sybil (interview), "How to survive (practically) anything," *Psychology Today,* Vol. 25, No. 1, January–February 1992.

151 Kramer, Peter, *Listening to Prozac.* New York: Penguin Books, 1993.

153 Szasz, Thomas, "Mental illness is still a myth," *Society,* Vol. 31, No. 4, May–June 1994.

156 Szasz, Thomas, *The Therapeutic State.* Buffalo: Prometheus Books, 1984.

158 Raso, Jack, "Alternative healthcare, Ayurveda, and neo-Hinduism," *Nutrition Forum,* Vol. 11, No. 4, July–August 1994.

159 Chopra, Deepak, *Return of the Rishi.* Boston: Houghton Mifflin Co., 1988.

Chapter 7 How to Protect Yourself, and Those You Love, from Misdiagnosis

166 Walker, Sydney, III, *Psychiatric Signs and Symptoms Due to Medical Problems.* New York: Charles C. Thomas, 1967.

167 Watterson, Kathryn, *The Safe Medicine Book.* New York: Ballantine Books, 1988.

168   Twerski, Abraham, *Who Says You're Neurotic?* Englewood Cliffs, NJ: Prentice-Hall, Inc., 1984.

174   Gross, David A., Extein, Irl, and Gold, Mark S., "The psychiatrist as physician," in *Medical Mimics of Psychiatric Disorders,* Irl Extein and Mark S. Gold, eds. Washington DC: American Psychiatric Press, Inc., 1986.

175   Kra, Siegfried, *Aging Myths: Reversible Causes of Mind and Memory Loss.* New York: McGraw-Hill Book Co., 1986.

180   Blue Cross statistics from *The Doctor's People,* Vol. 2, No. 9, 1989.

181   Kirk, Stuart, and Kutchins, Herb, *The Selling of DSM: The Rhetoric of Science in Psychiatry.* New York: Aldine de Gruyter, 1992.

182   Goldstein, Jay, *Could Your Doctor Be Wrong?* New York: Pharos Books, 1991.

184   Faust, D., Hart, K., and Guilmette, T. J., "Pediatric malingering: the capacity of children to fake believable deficits on neuropsychological testing," *Journal of Consulting and Clinical Psychology,* Vol. 58, 1988.

185   Dawes, Robyn, *House of Cards: Psychology and Psychotherapy Built on Myth.* New York: The Free Press, 1994.

185   Jagger, C., Clarke, M., Anderson, J., and Battcock, T., "Misclassification of dementia by the Mini-Mental State Examination—are education and social class the only factors?" *Age and Ageing,* Vol. 21, No. 6, November 1992.

186   Inlander, Charles B., Levin, Lowell, S., and Weiner, Ed, *Medicine on Trial.* Englewood Cliffs, NJ: Prentice-Hall Press, 1988.

189   *The New Harvard Guide to Psychiatry,* Armand M. Nicholi, Jr., ed. Cambridge, MA: Belknap Press, 1988.

192   Wolfe, Sidney, Fugate, Lisa, Hulstrand, Elizabeth, and Kamimoto, Laurie, *Worst Pills/Best Pills.* Washington, DC: Public Citizen Health Research Group, 1988.

192   Kra, Siegfried, *Aging Myths: Reversible Causes of Mind and Memory Loss.* New York: McGraw-Hill Book Co., 1986.

199   Bergin, Daniel M., *Drug Topics,* Vol. 134, No. 16, August 20, 1990.

202   Tupper, John, cited in Maggie Garb, "Can psychologists learn to prescribe?" *American Medical News,* Vol. 34, No. 8, 1991.

203   Maxmen, Jerrold, *The New Psychiatry.* New York: William Morrow and Co., 1985.

Chapter 8 "But I'm Not a Patient!"

207 Faust, David, and Ziskin, Jay, "The expert witness in psychology and psychiatry," *Science,* Vol. 241, July 1, 1988.

207 Robitscher, Jonas, *The Powers of Psychiatry.* Boston: Houghton Mifflin Co., 1980.

208 Doherty, Brian, "Unreasonable accommodations," *Reason,* Vol. 27, No. 4, August/September 1995.

209 Bovard, James, "The lame game," *American Spectator,* Vol. 28, No. 7, July 1995.

210 Topolnicki, Denise, Tritch, Teresa, and Gilbert, Beth, "The gulag of guardianship," *Money,* Vol. 18, No. 3, March 1989.

211 Kirk, Stuart A., and Kutchins, Herb, *The Selling of DSM: The Rhetoric of Science in Psychiatry.* New York: Aldine de Gruyter, 1992.

212 Herman, Stephen P., and Levy, Alan M., "Does peer review have a place in child custody evaluations?" *Children Today,* Vol. 18, No. 3, May–June 1989.

212 Chesler, Phyllis, *Mothers on Trial.* New York: McGraw-Hill, 1986.

214 Faust, David, and Ziskin, Jay, "The expert witness in psychology and psychiatry," *Science,* Vol. 241, July 1, 1988.

215 Dawes, Robyn, *House of Cards: Psychology and Psychotherapy Built on Myth.* New York: The Free Press, 1994.

216 Markman, Ronald, and Bosco, Dominick, *Alone with the Devil.* Garden City, NY: Doubleday, 1989.

219 Ullman, Joan, "I carried it too far, that's for sure," *Psychology Today,* Vol. 25, No. 3, May–June 1992.

220 Five-year study of "nonviolent" prisoners cited by Neuman, Elena, in "Abuse excuse goes on trial," *Insight on the News,* March 28, 1994.

222 Watzman, Nancy, and Saletan, William, "Marcus Welby, J.D.: when doctors become judges," *The New Republic,* April 17, 1989.

222 Szasz, Thomas, *The Therapeutic State.* Buffalo: Prometheus Books, 1984.

223 Brunner, H. G., Nelen, M., Breakefield, X. O., Ropers, H. H., and Oost, B. A. van, "Abnormal behavior associated with a point mutation in the structural gene for monoamine oxidase A," *Science,* Vol. 262, No. 5133, October 22, 1993.

223 Denno study cited in *Crime Times,* Vol. 1, No. 3, 1995.

223 Rosenbaum, Alan, and Hoge, Steven, "Head injury and marital aggression," *American Journal of Psychiatry,* Vol. 146, No. 8, August 1989.

224 Rosenbaum, Alan, Hoge, Steven K., Adelman, Steven K., Warnken, William J., Fletcher, Kenneth E., and Kane, Robert L., "Head injury in partner-abusive men," *Journal of Consulting and Clinical Psychology,* Vol. 62, No. 6, 1994.

224 Mark, V. H., and Ervin, F. R., *Violence and the Brain.* New York: Harper & Row, 1970.

Chapter 9 Where Do We Go from Here?

226 Torrey, E. Fuller, *The Death of Psychiatry.* Radnor, PA: Chilton Book Co., 1974.

228 For a more extensive discussion of clinical neuronal reductivism, see Walker, Sydney, III, "The parable of the elephant: exploring clinical reductivism," *Psychiatric Times,* September 1995.

228 Denny-Brown, Derek, personal communication, 1963.

229 "Pushing drugs to doctors," *Consumer Reports,* February 1992.

231 Szasz, Thomas, "Mental illness is still a myth," *Society,* Vol. 31, No. 4, May–June, 1994.

Index